PENGUIN BOOKS

# Letters to My Fanny

Cherry Healey is a television presenter, famous for her BBC3 documentaries covering topics including drinking, money, relationships, pregnancy and body image, and also for her science and food documentaries on BBC1 and BBC2.

# Letters to My Fanny

CHERRY HEALEY

PENGUIN BOOKS

PENGUIN BOOKS

UK | USA | Canada | Ireland | Australia

India | New Zealand | South Africa

Penguin Books is part of the Penguin Random House group of companies
whose addresses can be found at global.penguinrandomhouse.com

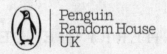

First published 2016

007

Text copyright © Cherry Healey, 2016

The moral right of the author has been asserted

Set in 12.5/16pt Garamond MT Std

Typeset in India by Thomson Digital Pvt Ltd, Noida, Delhi

Printed and bound in Great Britain by Clays Ltd, St Ives plc

A CIP catalogue record for this book is available from the British Library

B FORMAT ISBN: 978–1–405–91979–1

www.greenpenguin.co.uk

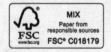

MIX
Paper from
responsible sources
FSC® C018179

Penguin Random House is committed to a
sustainable future for our business, our readers
and our planet. This book is made from Forest
Stewardship Council® certified paper.

This is for all the amazing women and men I've been inspired by and who have shared their passionate views with me over many bowls of nachos and vodka Diet Cokes. This is also for my wonderful mum who taught me how to listen and love and make a cracking lasagne, and for my daughter who I love so much that I wish I had a wider vocabulary to give it justice.

# Introduction

For my final dissertation at university I decided to write, voluntarily, about existentialism. My tutors advised against it but, because I had seen a really interesting talk on the subject, I felt it would be a good idea. Of course, ten thousand words later I was in a right pickle and had premature grey hairs. I vowed never, ever to write more than a hundred and forty characters in a row ever again.

And then for some reason that only the heavens understand and probably not even them, I decided to write a book. Perhaps it was a compulsive desire to impart my learnings to my daughter or perhaps it was because with two children and a busy job I just felt like I had too much free time. But I comforted myself that it would be a pretty short book: perhaps a stocking filler or something light to read whilst you're on the loo.

Then somehow I managed to write nearly a hundred thousand words. It was actually a bit like having a baby. At times I was swollen with ideas and thoughts. At other times I felt sick with nerves at the knowledge that my musings would be published on paper. And, like having a baby, it took a really flipping long time – especially as I spend most of my time chasing my actual babies around after their bath. But, finally, I have managed to push it out and it is now its own entity.

What follows is my own story. Not a lecture, not a manual, but my own personal experiences of being a woman.

There is still so much pressure on women in the twenty-first century to look and act a certain way. Like most women, I've felt these pressures every day from such a young age that I rarely stop to reflect on them.

The turning point for me was having the babies I mentioned above (the real ones, not the book baby). All of a sudden, I realized that my body was capable of something incredible – giving life to another human. But it also made me realize that my body was my own, to do what I wanted with. Want to create a baby? Yup, no biggie. Want to write a book? Well, it's just done that too. Want to run a marathon? Well . . . now that I know it can make your nipples bleed maybe I'll give that one a miss.

I'm not a feminist academic, but I do believe that if women want to speak out, they should feel free to, regardless of their qualifications. Progress takes all sorts of voices and perspectives and doesn't need correct iambic pentameter to be relevant. We shouldn't sit in silence on how we *really* feel about ourselves, our fears, passions, work, money, love, our body.

So this book is a love letter, to my body. In fact, it's several letters – to every part from my brain to my belly. After years of hating it, I've realized that it deserves some well overdue TLC. I hope you enjoy reading this. Except you, Mum and Dad. You can stop reading. Now. It's for the best.

# 1. Letter to My Fanny: Orgasms, Sex, Periods

*Dear . . . um, Dear . . . er . . . OK, let's go with 'Fanny'.*

*Sorry, bad start. It's just hard to know what to call you. Which is a bit of a giveaway. 'Fanny' sounds so childish, but then 'vagina' doesn't feel friendly enough. I've called you so many things to get a laugh: minge, growler, hairy falafel, pink trifle (I know, I'm sorry); the list is endless and becomes even better – or worse – after a few drinks. I should probably apologize for the name-calling. Soz. I also need to address how badly I have neglected you. I'm not entirely sure why, but I am slightly nervous of you. You have been a bit of an unknown entity. And even at the age of thirty-four, you still are.*

*Perhaps this is a result of being at a girls-only boarding school from the ages of ten to eighteen. However, I suspect it is probably a mix of many different things: being English; being from a family that didn't talk about sex; having three brothers; being more comfortable in a jester's role than a sexy-time role; idolizing Sigourney Weaver / Ellen Ripley from* Alien. *But, dear long-suffering Fanny, the time for reconciliation is here. You have given me an incredible bite-her-bottom-cute daughter and now an equally lovely son who smells like biscuits, and I think you deserve some appreciation.*

*So thank you, a million times thank you, for the good times, the bad times and the ugly times. I promise never to trim you with*

1

*scissors whilst texting ever again — that was callous and we both*
*suffered — and I wish someone had told me that rushed, inexperi-*
*enced self-waxing can result in your lady garden looking like a*
*toddler has tried to papier-mâché it with candle wax. I could have*
*done without the repeated cystitis, if I'm honest. But no biggie,*
*definitely my fault and rectified now that I've learned the magical*
*lady trick of going for a wee after sex — which as far as I'm*
*concerned should be on the curriculum — and always staying*
*hydrated, just not with sangria.*

*I hope that now I am gently entering my fourth decade we can*
*be friends. Maybe even more than friends. I wonder whether, after*
*writing this, we'll be on intimate terms rather than dancing around*
*each other like two suspicious street dogs.*

*I hope so.*

*All my love,*
*Cherry x*


## Orgasms

So, people, let us discuss sexual pleasure and maybe even
our love apparatus.

Um. Hang tight.

This is a touch awkward.

Not something we talk about all that freely, given how
modern and liberal and emancipated we all think we are.

I think part of the problem for me has been my discomfort with being overtly sexual; I'm far more at home being silly. I usually go for Halloween costumes that involve boiler suits and blood-splattered make-up rather than 'sexy witch' or 'seductive vampiress'. I'm particularly thinking of the time I went to a fresher's party as Eminem with a chainsaw made from a cardboard box and chicken wire. I did not pull.

I think I first became aware of my fanny at the age of seven or eight when I was given *The Body Book* by Claire Rayner, which sweetly explains the mechanics of the body, from how the brain works to eating and doing a poo (I have never looked at nuts and raisins in the same way since). And, of course, reproduction – or 'Making New People' as it was called. My brother and I must have read this book a hundred times and we knew, even in our innocence, that it was a bit 'rude'. It now sits proudly on my bookshelf, waiting until my children are old enough to know about the birds and the bees (and nuts and raisins).

My favourite extract reads: 'When boys and girls are almost grown-up, some important bits of them start to grow. These are the baby-making bits . . . When a man and a woman want to make a baby, the man's penis stops being floppy and hanging down. It stands to attention. This is a special grown-up way of loving someone very much. It is the most loving sort of cuddle there is for grown-ups.'

Despite this promising start, I then stopped thinking about my fanny for a few years and instead focused on learning Michael Jackson routines in my bedroom, wearing satin waistcoats decorated with large multicoloured diamonds of leftover curtain material (lovingly handmade by my mum), velvet leggings and loafers, and thinking about what was for tea. I do remember enjoying the trip home from school via the bakery, which involved driving over humps in the road. That was when I first realized there was some kind of 'special' action going on down there. I'm not sure what I enjoyed more, the chocolate-dipped flapjack or the humped bridge.

The next encounter with my lady-area was so monu-mentally, Mexican-wave-inducingly mind-blowing that it should really have been the beginning of an utterly joyful sexual adventure. But it was in fact a long time until I connected what had happened to actual sexual activity. I remember it so vividly I can pretty much recount every detail. I was about ten years old and had gone with my parents to stay with some family friends. I felt very grown-up as my bedroom had a double bed and an en-suite bathroom – my first experience of such finery. Before dinner, excited to use the facilities (I do love to make use of the facilities), I ran myself an enormous bath and hopped in, excited to try the extensive and fancy-sounding products (what is this luxury item? Badedas?!). And then, innocent as the day was bright, I cranked up the power shower and set myself free from the tower of bubbles I had created. And, entirely by accident, suffered a direct hit in the middle of my fanny. *BOOM!*

I wasn't sure if I was dying or having a stroke, or perhaps some sort of spiritual experience, but I was completely and utterly gobsmacked. I remember sitting on the edge of the bath staring into oblivion. I couldn't fathom what had just happened. It wasn't exactly 'BOOM!' but more like a motorbike revving up and going from nought to sixty in six seconds, which isn't far off Boom Speed. I was slightly scared – was it normal for people's fannies to explode? It took about five minutes to gather myself and go into the bedroom, where I sat on the bed and stared some more, trying to make sense of what had just happened. Perhaps I was more naive than other kids my age but I had no idea what an orgasm was – this was before the internet existed (*how did we live?*) and when I had watched *When Harry Met Sally* I thought the café scene was Meg Ryan trying to mimic someone dying. All I had to go on was the information supplied by *The Body Book*. At no point did the gentle words or cosy illustrations mention *this*. The book had told me all about nuts and raisins and why a man's willy stands to attention. But it had not revealed this magical secret of the female body. Why, oh why, would you exclude something as GIGANTICALLY, HUMONGOUSLY important as this? This is surely *the* moment where someone comes of age (biting my hand not to exercise the very obvious pun here) and there should be a bit of a heads-up, no?

I got dressed in a daze and went downstairs for dinner. (It was chicken pie and peas – as I said, I remember that day like it was yesterday.) Of course the minute I saw my parents I felt like they somehow knew what had just taken place – my cheeks were still flushed and the colour of a raspberry. We sat and ate our pie and peas and the grown-ups chatted about the price of houses and I anxiously hoped my vagina would not explode again or fall off under the table for the dog to eat. The whole experience was so shocking that it was about three years until I ventured back into that area.

I have, thankfully, learned a little more about orgasms since then and I am still learning every day. I have learned that there are lots of different types of orgasm. There are loud ones, deep ones, shallow ones, clitoral ones, love-tunnel ones, bum ones, squeaky ones, squirty ones and shouty ones. Like driving a car, in my younger years I would start the engine and see where it took me, but as I've become more practised I am starting to know which route to take to get to a certain place. If you know what I mean (everyone knows what I mean). I did realize the other day that, although my friends and I are open with each other, we have never had a graphic conversation about how we achieve different types of orgasm. Which is both completely understandable and a bit silly. There are perhaps one trillion and twelve food progammes and bloggers telling us how to experience different types of edible delight (I love them all), yet most of us, with a few lucky exceptions, live a life where we find our way to sexual completion (an amazing phrase I heard recently from a medical professional) almost completely blind. Some may say that porn is sexual education but I can safely say from the porn I have watched it is the Antichrist of learning about female orgasms.

So where do we learn about how to have a good/better/multiple/really lovely/give me a minute to return to earth female orgasm/s? Well. It's not parents (I'm imagining that conversation and I think a part of me just died). It's not porn, unless panting for forty minutes like you're in a spin class and staring coldly into the middle distance whilst touching el clitoris for fifteen seconds counts. And it's not school – although I'd much rather learn about this than how to make a quiche. It's probably not from the internet – when I type in 'Women and Orgasms' the first hit is for an article in *Men And Fitness* magazine talking about how to 'Get her off every time!' and the second is from a medical site stating that, because women don't need to orgasm in order to conceive, doctors don't rate the importance of female orgasm highly. This explains so much.

It is, I am sure for most women, trial and error. And thank goodness we now live in a culture/time where we are not only allowed to do it, but we are starting to admit it openly. In times gone by sexual desire and orgasm were considered symptoms of hysteria, a medical condition sometimes resulting in admission to an insane asylum or a hysterectomy or electric shock treatment. I know this sounds morbid but I do sometimes think about that when

I am mooching about casually shopping in Coco de Mer. The lack of freedom for the women who lived before us is almost unfathomable.

The more I researched the link between hysteria and women's sexual self, the more I found myself struggling to read the words in front of me. It is no coincidence that the removal of a woman's womb, a hysterectomy, is similar in sound and look to the word 'hysteria'. Not to get too far into a territory that I have little to no knowledge about, but it's believed that this stems as far back as the fourth and fifth centuries BC, when Plato compared a woman's uterus to a living creature 'blocking passages, obstructing breathing and causing disease'. Can we have a moment here to remember that he was, and still is, respected as one of the great thinkers of all time? That kind of information really helps me to understand why it has been and continues, for many, to be a man's world. Women sound creepy, unpredictable and dangerous. It also clearly explains why men can delight in, talk about and laugh casually about the frequency and preferred style of masturbating, whereas women, historically, might have been taken away in a van and locked up. Vibrators were initially invented as a way to cure hysteria as doctors believed they released the build-up of female semen, which could turn venomous, thus causing hysteria, if not released through orgasm. Wow. I shed a tear for all of those women who were put through all of those traumatic treatments. Sitting here now, with so much sexual education at my fingertips, and the ability to freely learn about how my body works with a rainbow of toys and techniques, I catch a glimpse of how far we've come. But we're not there yet.

One of the many gifts given to us by the universe is the multiple orgasm. I have had a few. At the moment they happen by surprise but I wish to one day learn how to exercise them on demand because they feel quite nice. To say the least. It's a bit like when a smart restaurant serves you a surprise and free bonus pre-starter starter. I haven't yet learned how to do it in the presence of another human being because, like playing the piano, I do my best work in this area without the pressure of an audience. But, as we all know, practice makes perfect, so I will continue to practise privately because it's extremely enjoyable and also helps when it comes to the big recital.

Multiple orgasms and female ejaculation are both, according to expects, achievable for most women but, according to my friends, experienced very rarely. I wonder if, in the same way that I read about women being treated for hysteria with disbelief, my daughter's daughter's generation will look back and feel amazed that women accepted a sexual life of no orgasms (ten per cent according to studies), fake orgasms (yeah, I've done that), single orgasms and dry orgasms (or whatever the opposite to an ejaculationary orgasm is known as – answers on a postcard). I am sure that the sexual liberation of women will continue on like a Duracell-powered rabbit and women will come to know their bodies better than a black cab knows The Knowledge.

# Sex

Which leads me on to sex. I'm writing this with trepidation because even though I have made a pretty candid documentary about losing your virginity, in which I told my story in broad brushstrokes, it's different committing it to paper. Television programmes cometh and goeth, blink and you'll miss them, but with print it can be read, reread and quoted with much more ease, and therefore taken out of context. I wonder if I'm particularly nervous about broaching this subject because of the public reaction to the documentary. The part that drew the media's attention was when I accompanied a seventeen-year-old girl to get a bikini wax. Yup. This was an appointment she had made herself, with her parents' approval, to prepare for a holiday where she planned to lose her virginity, also approved by her parents and something that they had discussed together in an open and mature way. This, of course, is the antithesis of what most of us experience when we're younger, when we painstakingly hide our sexual activities from our parents and dive head first into a situation that we had not really thought about or prepared for and subsequently end up regretting.

In the end this girl went on holiday, had a fumble with a boy and decided that she wanted to wait and have sex with someone she loved. But for some reason this hit the headlines and, as I remember, even made it on to the news in Australia. It was bonkers. I really did not understand why this wasn't being heralded as a fabulous example of an open, honest relationship between a teenage girl and her parents. Surely if we really want our teenagers to better avoid unprotected sex, or sex before they're ready, or secretive behaviour, then this family and this situation was a shining role model for a healthy attitude to talking about sex?

But what I found really surprising was that the media completely ignored the most shocking moment in the whole programme. I had also interviewed some young teenagers in a park in Wales (I remember it vividly because I thought my face was going to fall off from frostbite) and they told me that they never used condoms. Ever. Because they 'break the atmosphere'. And the girls told me that they didn't complain because they were getting attention from the boys and most certainly weren't going to risk scaring one away by demanding he wear a condom. Some of the boys had lost their virginity at twelve and were already, at the age of sixteen, into double figures. When I asked them what they would do if a girl became pregnant, or if they caught an STD, they just shrugged. A few of them had had chlamydia but felt it wasn't much of a biggie; lots of people have it and are fine, they said. I explained to the boys that if they passed this on to a girl it could make her infertile, but I could see that my words had little or no impact.

And I wasn't even that surprised because I can remember being a teen (increasingly hard and, yes, things are very different for teens now). But I *can* remember feeling invincible, and I sensed a similar attitude from the teens I was interviewing. Some of the things I did when I was younger were so dangerous and done in such a cavalier way that it makes my skin hurt just remembering them. The future felt so, so far away and the consequences were not something we wasted our precious free time thinking about. Especially if there were boys and Malibu around. All I was concerned with was how quickly I could get drunk and if I was going to get a snog from a hot boy, both factors being inextricably entwined. Having never had a conversation with an adult about sex and only gleaning random pieces of information from my equally fumbling-in-the-dark teenage friends, I had absolutely no game plan if things progressed to actual sex. My focus was on the thrill of the chase and the ten pounds in my pocket that I knew I should save for a bus fare and a sand-wich but would almost certainly be spent on cigarettes and chips.

It's an age-old problem: older people, who have made mistakes and felt the consequences, try to impart wisdom to young people who haven't yet felt consequences and therefore do not care about consequences. The older peo-ple then feel vexed by said young people when they don't listen, and then themselves feel frustrated when they remember that they were *exactly* the same when they were young. Of course, you can't live people's lives for them; part of the joy of growing up is experiencing the fear and excitement of life first-hand, discovering the subsequent consequences and then making your own assessment of the risks for the future. To try to take this away from young people is both futile and missing the point of existence. But at the same time it doesn't hurt to try to establish an open, shame-free, honest dialogue with people who might want to try banging because it seems (and they're bang on) really fun.

So anyway, here was a group of twelve- and thirteen-year-olds telling me all about their sexual adventures and on the one hand I'm thinking, *Wow, this is so shocking*, and on the other I'm remembering what I was like when I was younger. The seventeen-year-old girl I met making the documentary was so, so much more mature and thoughtful than I or many of my friends were at that age. She had consciously decided she was tired of waiting for the mythical 'one'; she wanted to go somewhere with a trusted group of friends and felt ready to break the ice, so to speak. She had protection, awareness and a plan for how to keep everything safe if action presented itself. So for the papers to get their knickers in a twist about this particular story seemed, well, pretty crackers to me.

The more people I interviewed for the programme, the more I realized that for most of us this seminal moment is often a fumble in the dark, often painful and often fuelled by some kind of pineapple-flavoured spirit that is then vomited down the side of your friend's dad's car on the way home. But I also found out that, thankfully, the way you lose your virginity does not at all dictate your future sexual experiences. And, to be honest, in my particular case I would say that my sexual journey definitely got off on the wrong willy.

I was so keen to lose my virginity that I . . . sort of got a bit muddled. There is a fine line between enthusiasm and confusion, and that is definitely where I was. I've always believed that losing your virginity is like becoming pregnant – you can't do it in half measure. Except that I managed to break my own rule. I'm sure there were many reasons for such haste to pop my cherry but I sometimes wonder if it was the Corridor Chat that gave me my motivation. At my all-girls boarding school, in the evenings we would congregate in the corridor, settle on Marmite-stained biohazard beanbags, eat an entire loaf of Nutella-slathered toast (each), make tea and chat. It was a mixture of therapy and sex education in a DIY café environment. There was even a whiteboard, which became extremely useful when trying to describe a particularly complicated piece of biology. And, because we were at boarding school for seven years with very limited access to television, stories from our holidays and weekends at home were like gold dust.

One summer my wonderful mum took me and some friends to a seaside town for a sun, surfing and Mr Whippy fest. Of course as fifteen-year-olds we had an entirely different agenda. During the day, my friend and I would boogie-board, eat hot chips and cold ice cream and listen to Green Day on our portable CD players, which obviously ended up with sand in them because the CD era was designed by people who never went to the beach or even outside without white gloves on. After the sun went down and we were red with burn and blue with cold, we'd have a good scrub, put on our velvet leggings, Doc Martens and head out to meet 'friends'. By friends I mean random strangers who had also told their beloved and trusting parents that they were meeting 'friends'. And boy oh boy were we friendly. In those magical days we all had fake IDs, which pubs actually accepted without running our DNA through the national database. All the pub staff wanted to know was that they could proclaim innocence if the police turned up, as they often did. This always seemed like a pointless exercise to me as we were clearly very underage, but as long as we had our Tippexed and Sellotaped piece of plastic we could drink as much Archers and lemonade as we could fit into our pubescent bodies. And if you were fortunate enough to have a friend that had enjoyed a growth spurt, facial hair, good clothes and/or money, then you could even get shots.

On one particularly fun night I remember arriving at the most infamous pub, the Mariners, and noticing the excellently large number of hot 'friends'. We diligently set about the hard work of getting hammered on not much money and the subtle game of eye contact, no eye contact, pretend-we-don't-see-their eye contact, pray for eye contact and so on. At some point I must have made actual, real contact with the person I had made 'friends' with that evening but I have no memory of it. All I remember is suddenly being under a boat with him on the beach and hands being everywhere. (For those that are thinking *Her pooooor parents*, I assure you I have requested that they don't read this. They have probably already heard worse on my documentaries but obviously I am moving to Ulan Bator the minute this is published, just in case.)

So here I am, under a boat, drunk, and as always just going with it without much thought. This is where a plan could have been useful, but there we go. I had no plan; I had hormones and the need for an exciting story for Corridor Chat. I know that sounds ridiculous but remember the last time you went out for a work do/hen party/ any party and did something crazy? Be honest now – did you proceed partly because you knew it would make an amazing story? Exactly.

Right. I'm under a boat, I'm fifteen, and this boy was getting involved. At some point his willy was near me and maybe on my leg and stuff and *perhaps* went north and . . . that was it, I assumed I *had* 'lost it'. And by 'it', I don't mean my tights (although I had lost those and they were new from Tammy Girl, so that was very annoying). I can't remember how I got out from under the boat or what was said or what his name was (like, err, totally irrelevant) but I do remember *running* up to my friend and proclaiming in a drunk whisper (i.e. shouting) that I had just had *SEX*. Friend that she was, her eyes popped out of her head and we knew that we now had something to talk about for the next year. I had taken one for the team.

Six months later I met a beautiful boy who also happened to be a beautiful person and I started to experience what people call 'feelings'. For some unknown reason he didn't mind my spots, puppy fat, braces or bad shoes. In fact, he seemed to really, really like me. I found this all very suspicious.

We spend time together (never under a boat), we meet each other's parents, and we eventually kiss at the back of a bus to the applause of our friends who are exhausted by the painfully shy dance of avoidance we do every time we are together. Things move slowly because he seems to like actually talking to me. I start to be myself around him and the sillier I am, the more he seems to like me. I have a small nuclear revelation that perhaps boys want more than somewhere to put their fingers (I'm sorry). No one is more surprised than me that nine months later we are still together, he still seems to really like me and we are actual girlfriend and boyfriend. From where I am now, I can see that it was very sweet but at the time it didn't feel sweet; it felt cool and grown-up. And you can imagine the joy this brought the Corridor discussion panel.

And again, in the interest of everyone's sanity, I won't linger too much on the gory details of our first time – although I suppose, to some people, I have already crossed that line on national television. Anyway, at this point I had realized that my experience with Boat Boy wasn't quite what I had thought at the time. As my memory returned (in that horrible post-night-out cold wave) and my knowledge of sex grew, I had to admit to myself that I might have been talking bollocks. But I comforted myself with the silver lining that at least this meant that I *hadn't* lost my virginity with a random name-less boy who had bleached-blond gel-crisp hair under a boat in the middle of nowhere, in the middle of the night, with sand up my crack. So here I was again, like a virgin, wanting to be touched for the very second time, although it was in fact the first time, kind of, and – oh God, it's all so confusing being teenager.

And the gods of sex must have been looking down on me and decided that I'd had my fair share of grubby encounters because the first time with my boyfriend was lovely. I was staying at his house and we'd been talking all night in the spare room where I was staying. And with no fanfare or drama we decided to have sex. (I don't know why but I struggled to write that sentence. There is some-thing too cold about 'have sex', but 'make love' is beyond hideous and 'do it' too crude. Feel free to tweet me if you have any good alternatives.) Here's what I remember. We had a condom, it was getting light outside and it hurt like a mother-trucker. He was wonderful and caring and tried to make it hurt as little as possible but I remember tears rolling down my cheeks and biting my lip so hard it made a mark. So it happened and then we talked more and then went to sleep. It was calm and painful but not scary and mostly happy and, thankfully, the polar opposite to my first nearly-time.

The next day I felt so, so strange. But good strange. I went home and had an almost out-of-body conversation with my mum, *convinced* that she could tell. I'm sure this is a fairly common reaction but I felt like everyone I spoke to knew.

Nearly twenty years later, I am surprised I remember it so clearly. I think it's highly unlikely that someone's first time will feel really great (well, for girls anyway) but I do think if you a) feel happy and comfortable with the other person, b) are sober enough to remember it, and c) use protection, it counts as a win.

So that was my fanny's first proper contact with a willy and I'd say it was pretty great.

What is good sex? What is bad sex? How can you tell if you're doing it right? How adventurous should you be/ are you allowed to be? What is an acceptable fantasy and when does it become something to keep quiet about?

I have learned a few things during my sexual encounters but one of the most surprising moments along the way was when I discovered the vital skill of fluid management. Have you ever seen even the sniff of a mention of human fluid in a movie sex scene? The romantic happening just happens and everyone gets out of bed and pulls on their pants and off they go to get on with their daily activities. I would like to see a film in which, after imparting his human fluid unto his lady friend, the guy dashes off to get a flannel or a handful of loo paper whilst the girl skilfully crosses her legs to prevent leakage or where, particularly exhausted after exerting herself greatly during the coitus act, she decides she can't be bothered to get up and uses the sheet. It's laundry day anyway. Fluid management comes as a surprise when you start having sex. It's also a shock, and something useful to be aware of, when about an hour after the act of sexual intercourse some of the man love comes out without a huge amount of notice. It's a little like wetting yourself a little bit but with a sense of pride. At the beginning stages of someone's sexual life, when it's all fumbly and embarrassing anyway, it would be hugely helpful to know that this was totally normal and that even girls in the films who have perfect hair and smell like vanilla would also sometimes experience leakage whilst getting their lunch in the canteen. Sex is beautiful and wonderful and fun and messy and human and sometimes requires a flannel on standby.

Another surprise is that sometimes sex happens when your period is also happening. I was also surprised and delighted to find out that some guys don't care. A little like the flannel, something as basic as a towel can solve a problem like Maria. It all depends on how comfortable you/he/they are about human functions. I would say that it's more common for people to not want to engage in sexy time while the painters are in, so if you find someone who has accepted this is a natural and miraculous part of being a woman, and only requires a little bit of foresight to overcome, then give them a big kiss. I've also learned that, in lieu of a spare towel, the shower is a great location.

Speaking of periods and flannels . . .

## Periods

WAIT, wait, before you hurl the book to the floor, I BEG you . . . to ponder upon how little there has been written on this magical subject.

Yes, magical. For something so monumentally important and wonderful and life-giving, we almost never celebrate this incredible occurrence (oh, don't tell me you're squeamish – we watch nature programmes where spiders eat their own spawn without blinking and this is far, far neater). I know the advertisements make us think that periods are so heinous we need to use euphemisms such as 'that time' and use strange blue fluid that like looks like a WKD being poured on to a nappy but without them we would not be here. And anyway, in an age when some people think it's OK to text each other pictures of mammary glands and willies and whatever body part has recently been buffed I think it should be OK to talk about this.

Periods are a little like rain: we are annoyed when they show up but worried when they don't. We take them for granted, give them unpleasant but quite funny names (the curse, blob, the paper cut, the crime scene) and try to hide them altogether. I recently hosted a debate about why so many women have period shame and most of the audience admitted they went to great efforts to hide any sign of their period, including hiding a tampon under their jumper if they're walking through the office to the loo or preferring to wrap a used tampon in a roll of loo paper and hide it in their handbags rather than leave it in a boyfriends' bathroom bin or making sure that they are using the self-service till if they need to buy more. I've done all of these things many times.

I'm not suggesting we should wear badges notifying people when we're 'on', but I think it's unfair that periods are only associated with negativity: bad moods, swelling and fanny admin. Compare them to Glastonbury – we predominantly think about that festival with such national love and awe, whereas we could easily associate it with mud, queuing and stinky Portaloos. Periods need Glastonbury's PR team. Maybe the ad campaign could be 'They're bloody great.'

Ask most parents what it's like to have kids and they'll roll their eyes and talk about sleepless nights, purée and wipes. But take them to a quiet corner and their eyes will well up with tears of joy and, if you're really unlucky, they'll bring out their iPhone and show you a slide show of twenty-five different-but-the-same photographs of little Billy Bob on the swings (two is enough; *three is more than enough*). They'll also probably tell you that they're expecting, or would like, another child. Which might lead you to the conclusion that they are, in fact, absolutely loving parenthood. And you'd mostly be right. And, gentlewomen and excellent men, this is all thanks to the wonder that is The Period.

I spent most of my early teens wishing, praying that it would start and then, because it was how people talked about it, the minute it appeared I moaned about it. I can remember when it first happened to a friend of mine – I was eleven and on holiday with my best friend Lucy. There were three notable things about this holiday:

1. It was a cider-tasting holiday and it was the first time I got properly drunk and it was organized by her cool dad who had a cool beard.
2. It was the first time I wore denim shorts and I had just inherited my brother's Doc Martens boots and they were four sizes too big but I LOVED them, even though they made me look like Minnie Mouse and not in a good way.
3. Lucy started her period whilst we were climbing rocks on the beach and I remember it clearly because she went and became a woman without consulting me, her bezzie mate.

Hot on her heels, two years later, I got my first period. I was elated. Finally I had something to do with my prematurely stocked drawer of sanitary pads. I was ready to become a woman. It was, however, a huge anticlimax. My first period was less of a rite of passage, more of a reddish pant mark. Nevertheless I shared this gleefully with my fellow gossip-starved boarding-school friends and took advice on the best course of action. Obviously, ever over-keen to be a fully fledged adult, I was armed and ready with a tampon, but was advised against it by my wiser not-a-girl-not-yet-a-woman friends. Instead, I was told I should stop spending my precious pocket money on a drawer-full of snazzy-looking pads and instead I should become familiar with the crap range of sanitary pads in the school nurse's office as they were free and it meant you would always have an excuse for a little potter through the school midway through a particularly boring physics class. They ranged from long 'n' thick to walk-like-a-cowboy. As someone keen on sport this just didn't work for me – you try doing a cartwheel with a sleeping bag shoved down your Spandex gym knickers. If you finished the day without half of it scrunched into your bum crack and the other half dissolved into a strange mulch inside your pants you were one lucky lady-girl.

So, impatient from pad-induced chafing, I advanced quickly on to the real McCoy. Not as notable perhaps as losing one's virginity but clearly, to my fourteen-year-old self, worthy of a little diagram in my diary. Yes, I was so intrigued by the mechanics of tampons that it inspired art.*

---

* It's well worth a Google, if only for the woman who recently painted a portrait of Donald Trump using her own period blood.

I had sourced a packet of tampons from an older girl at school in an exchange so covert and slick you'd have thought we were dealing crack. A few things made me nervous about tampons. Firstly, they came with a fold-out instruction manual thicker than the nurses' sani pad. Secondly, I had seen an episode of *Casualty* where a girl left one up her lady area and became very, very unwell (i.e. toxic shock syndrome, which is a real thing but, as long as they're changed regularly, not something to be as paranoid about as I was). And thirdly, it is undoubtedly a brilliant but extremely weird invention.

However, having read the instruction booklet (including the terrifying possible side effects) word for word, I marched forward unto womanhood. One weekend, home from school in the privacy of our family bathroom, I took another turn towards becoming an adult. As you can imagine I was wide-eyed, excited and extremely careful when inserting a foreign object into my personage. For the following twenty-four hours I walked with a very deliberate light step, sure that at any minute the current tampon would fall out on to the floor and become my new Worst Teen Moment Ever of All Time (more on this later). But thankfully my first tampon stayed put and I happily waved goodbye to sanitary pads for ever and once again I had a whole new topic to share with the Corridor.

I'm probably waxing lyrical about periods because, as I'm writing this, I haven't actually had one for a while (half of this book was written whilst I was up the duff and the other after I'd given birth – I will try not to jump around too much). They say that absence makes the heart grow fonder and, thanks to pregnancy, I have had a little distance from the awkward handbag tampon fumbling, uncomfortable sanitary-pad scrunching and the occasional quick-as-a-ninja sheet change in response to a surprisingly heavy night. If you want to see a magic trick, see a woman disguise the evidence of an unexpected period, particularly in the presence of a new 'beau': Superman would struggle to get a wash on quicker. Or how about the stressful faff of trying to dispose of a sanitary pad when visiting someone's house who doesn't have a bin in their loo?

It's strange not to 'have' your period after it's been such a regular occurrence for over twenty years. Hmm, I'm not entirely sure why I put quotations around 'have', but it's so formal. Like 'I'm having a poo' is a silly phrase because it's such a formal statement for something funny. 'Having' goes with 'meetings' and 'dry white wine' and 'filling at the dentist'. It does not go with sex or periods. But I also don't like the phrases 'I'm *on* my period' or 'I'm currently menstruating, thank you very much' or 'the painters are in, don't you know?' For a country with such a planet-shaping language we are seriously lacking in some key areas.

So here *is* my Worst Teen Moment Ever of All Time. It makes me laugh to remember it but at the time I was *mortified*. I have an amazing male friend who I've been really close to since I was twelve. He is a joy, a funny mix between a real blokey bloke (i.e. he squirms when asked how he is 'feeling') and an incredibly intelligent, witty, hilarious, genuine gem. But definitely someone you go and play pool with and not someone – *really* not someone – to discuss periods with, or even mention them in any way whatsoever. One night, after burning a hole in our fake IDs at a pub that did not care a fig about teenage drinkers, I crashed with him at his parents' house round the corner. You've obviously raced ahead to the punchline already and, yes, I period-ed all over his bed. Oh God, I can feel the mortification all over again. I remember waking up in the morning and thinking, *No, no, no, no, no, no!* And then seeing the damage and thinking, *Oh shit, of all the places in the whole world, why, why, why?* And it wasn't a spot, or a smear – it was a stream, a surge, a superfluity. And, only millimetres away, sleeping soundly (we were sharing a bed but all very innocently) was my friend, unaware that I was having cardiac arrest over the increasingly large situation. Of course I went into panic mode and of course I tried to clean it up myself and of course that was a huge mistake. I assessed the extent of the problem and it was bad – the blood was all over my legs and my shorts and the sheets and I had to contort myself like a giraffe exiting a sports car in order to avoid spreading it further. And then, out of the bed and friend still asleep, I made a snap judgement. After shoving almost an entire loo roll between my legs, I then took one of the lovely, pristine, big white towels from the lovely, pristine, big white bathroom and made it damp under the tap. I then tried to clear up the blood. I know, I know: terrible, terrible sweat-inducing plan. I just spread it around further and made the towel look like it had been tie-dyed and got it all over the duvet cover in the process. This is all whilst desperately trying not to wake up my friend as the thought of having to deal with his horrified reaction was just too much to bear. So on I went, quiet as a mouse, making things worse and ruining yet another beautiful fluffy white towel. I finally accepted that there was nothing I could do and I would have to bite the bullet and go and tell The Mum.

I found his mother in the kitchen and, as I painfully explained what had happened, I accepted that she would never want to see me again, I would have to pay for the damage and I had essentially terminated my friendship with her son. But, because she is fabulous, she could see the agony in my face and brushed off this *earth-shatteringly* terrible life event as though someone had spilt a cup of tea. And, now I'm older and less easily mortified, I can see she was bang on. She casually said it was no problem and helped me flee. I think it took a good few weeks to see my friend again and a few months to look him in the eye, in case he could see into my soul and see what had happened. I have never asked my male friend whether he was aware of what happened but, by the end of writing this book, I promise I will have worked up the courage to have that conversation with him.

That was my first experience in period humiliation. As a teenager I absolutely, intrinsically knew within my bones that it was NOT OK to laugh with boys about periods. Nowadays girls can joke *reasonably* comfortably about farts but we cannot, making a safe generalization I think, laugh about a particularly fierce period day in the presence of boys without being faced with expressions of disgust. I wonder sometimes if we make a rod for our own sore backs. Are boys uncomfortable about this subject because we hide it from them? Or do we hide it from them because they are uncomfortable? I do wonder if we'll ever live in a world where we can say casually, 'Gosh, I am menstruating like a mother-trucker today, anyone got any spare big pants?' Half the population of our glorious globe menstruate and I think it's about time we were able to come out of the closet about this. It's nothing to be ashamed of – quite the opposite: we have to deal with some very annoying faff around it and I believe we do this with incredible ingenuity, grace and elegance – and we should not feel like it's our dirty secret.

I have been married for six years and I think the first time my husband saw one of my tampons was when I gave one to my toddler to play with (they make excellent emergency toys, FYI). He has seen me post-Caesarean in knee-high thrombosis socks and hospital-issue mesh pants, with a huge freshly stitched belly scar and catheter, hobbling to the loo like a pensioner orc, and yet *still* I would be so very, utterly embarrassed if he ever walked in on me dealing with a period.

It was only when I was thirty-one, after the birth of my daughter, that I really, really understood – and therefore appreciated – their function. Having been slightly blown off the face of the planet by how excellent my daughter was, I thought it might be very amazing to have another pop at it. And that's when I fully realized that the key to this was my periods. After being without them during pregnancy and then for a few months whilst I was breast-feeding and my body gathered its thoughts, I realized I really needed my periods to pay a visit. It's not that I missed the faff, but I suddenly appreciated their presence.

All hail the mighty period. All hail the wonderful miracle that is the Fanny.

# 2. Letter to My Hands: Fingering, Masturbation, Writing

*Darling Hands,*

*How do I love thee? Let me count the ways. And, thanks to you, I am able to. Yes, at thirty-four I still count using my fingers. I only wish I had more of them or was a monkey and was able to use my toes (my toes are almost long enough – I know, hot).*

*Without you I wouldn't be able to do the thing that propels me into ecstasy, that makes my eyes roll into the back of my head and takes me to another place: pick 'n' mix. In the past three decades, in pitch-black cinemas, you have foraged through countless paper tubs with applaudable dexterity. You are able to tell the difference between a fizzy and a virgin cola bottle, a chocolate or peanut raisin, a white or real mouse. That is no mean feat. You really know what you're doing and you have given me great pleasure.*

*There are so many things you do, and do so well. You shake, embrace, wave, point, communicate peace, flick the bird, text, swipe, click, nervously tap, pick, pray, clasp, catch, throw, rub, insert, repeat (and I'm not talking about pick 'n' mix this time).*

# Magic Hands

This chapter shouldn't really be called 'Hands', it should be called 'Claws', as that is what I have. When in motion, which is always, my 'hands' closely resemble the upper limbs of a T. rex. I think if I were to put a bag over my head and put tape over my mouth you would still know what I was trying to say through the power of The Claws (I bet some of my friends are reading this thinking how peaceful life would be if that were the case). I would now like to take this opportunity to apologize to all the directors who have tried to tame them, often unsuccessfully, and have had to subsequently frame them out. It's not stubbornness on my part, I promise – they have a life of their own.

Hands are a bit magic. There is a beautifully simple but powerful joy in holding someone's hand. That feeling of being on a third date with a boy you're crazy about (and you think, you hope with all of your being, that he might possibly be crazy about you) and you can feel something radiating between your hands like they are on fire and finally, God, *finally*, he grabs one and it feels like someone has just put a pin into the top of your head and popped you and the relief is physical, tangible.

The first time I wanted to desperately hold someone's hand was with my second kind-of boyfriend, Rodolf. I say 'kind-of' because, at that stage, a boyfriend was someone who was a) a boy, and b) a boy that had 'asked you out', often over the phone. (In the 'olden' days, boys had to call your family landline and speak to you with an actual voice rather than by text, and often via your parents in a shaky voice: 'Hi, Mr Healey, um, can I, um, speak to Cherry or something?', causing said parents to shout up the stairs, 'Cherry! Some boy wants to talk to you', resulting in all parties wishing someone would invent texting already.) And if you were waiting in the phone queue at boarding school (imagine something similar to the phone queue in a prison) then this very un-romantic encounter ended in an euphoric announcement to the whole room that 'HE'S ASKED ME OUT!' and that it was time to 'CRACK OPEN THE GOOD MARMITE!' Anything beyond this was a bonus.

Rodolf and I were fifteen and it was extremely exciting to have been 'asked out' as he was extremely cool and I was extremely not. And not only did he have everything that a fifteen-year-old girl required (cool trousers, a tenner and excellent hair – ginger dreadlocks, which trumped the second-best hairstyle that ever existed for boys: nineties curtains) but he was also a brilliant person. He was clever, kind and funny – a teenage slam-dunk.

After one particularly energetic session of kissing in the least dog-poo-infested part of the local park, and after laughing together about the ever-nearing flock of excited pigeons, I had my first sense of wanting to be someone's girlfriend, rather than just being grateful that another human being wanted to be my boyfriend. It was exciting to feel proactive rather than reactive, to have a relationship based on the joy of spending time together rather than just being a vehicle for a boy to achieve another sexual experience. I felt sure, I hoped with all of my heart, that Rodolf really did both fancy me and love hanging out with me, as was being demonstrated. And, as we walked along, wondering how to spend our remaining £3.75, I had the powerful desire for him to hold my hand. It didn't even cross my mind that I could initiate it – good God, no. Excuseeeee me but at what point in a Disney film, which was at the time my blueprint for romantic encounters (except *Dirty Dancing*, which had blown my tiny mind), did the princess EVER make the first move?

Anyway, back to me walking nervously next to Mr Cool, desperately searching for confirmation that he felt the same way, and something deeply romantic in me, perhaps primitive and natural or perhaps Disney brainwashing, wanted him to claim me in this simple but (to me) meaningful way. And, having decided that we should spend our remaining fortune on some dough balls and a Coke in Pizza Express, he took my hand and led me into the restaurant. And it was mind-blowingly fabulous. It was my first experience of enjoying the beautiful natural dynamic of male and female. I didn't mind being led, I didn't mind him asserting – quite the opposite – and at the time it didn't even cross my mind to question this.

Now I'm thirty-four and think a lot about the power balance between genders, the delicate balance between the male/female dynamic and of how to enjoy and embrace the feminine/masculine whilst not losing a sense of self-worth or power. But in this particular moment with Rodolf, it was just a simple, natural, comfortable and sexy gesture. And then we ate dough balls and laughed more about the crazy pigeons in the park.

I'd never really given much thought to the power of hands until one of them was taken – well, sort of – away from me. It's true that you don't know what you've got until it's gone. And strong functioning hands is definitely one of them. A few weeks after I had given birth to my first child, Coco, I had a brief but powerful lesson in hand appreciation. Whilst experiencing the expected sleep deprivation of a new parent, I developed the useful ability to pass out cold at any given nap opportunity, often falling asleep on my wrist, rather unhelpfully. And this happened night after night, gradually damaging my nerves and giving me something called carpal tunnel syndrome. This is fairly common during and after pregnancy, with sixty per cent of women experiencing the symptoms (tingling fingers, numbing, weak grip, swelling, aching around the wrist area) and is caused by a build-up of fluid, which puts pressure on the median nerve that runs down the arm. Yeah, that famous median nerve that everyone talks about.

So, when Coco was about six weeks old and the new-parent tiredness had really kicked in (like when you can't tie up your shoelaces and you start crying like your pet cat has been crushed by a car in front of you), I found that I would wake up with a strange floppy hand, like a puppet with no string. But I was far too busy/excited/confused by this very little, very new human being that had landed in my life to worry about something as silly as a floppy hand. I just tried to get on with things. I soon realized that I should *probably* get myself to the doctor when I was holding the baby in my left arm and switching on the kettle with my tongue. It was one of those moments when you are suddenly able to view yourself from the outside and realize that it's not OK to have to engage your elbow or tongue or toe when carrying out everyday activities like turning on the lights, pressing a doorbell or making a cup of tea. In one of my finest parenting moments, aware that I only had one functioning hand available, I decided to use my baby's head to turn off the bathroom light. Obviously she cried. Obviously I realized that was perhaps number one of the things not to do with a newborn's soft, not-yet-fused head. I would like to assure you that I was completely knackered and not at all malicious. That makes it better, yes?

It was, I told myself as I plopped a teabag into my mug using my teeth, time to visit a healthcare professional. It's not that I'm scared of the doctor, it's just that as a busy woman it's a bloody ball-ache, especially when you could be sleep, sleep, sleep, sleeping. However, because feeding and changing a baby is significantly harder one-handed, and because, more importantly, I like to text using both hands, I took myself off to see someone. Thankfully the solution was relatively simple and I was given a wrist harness with a metal splint (ensuring that my wrist and hand remained straight whilst I slept) and three sessions of physiotherapy. I love, with all of my heart, the NHS.

## Fingering

So finger appreciation comes in many forms and here is one that, if we're really going to get cosy and talk about tricky things, can't be omitted. In a word: fingering. (Yes, I did visibly cringe writing that – it is just one of those subjects that is inexplicably, astronomically, perhaps even globally, embarrassing.)

Here we go. I am tentatively, and with one eye closed due to the knowledge that my parents may read this (despite my requests to give this one/all of it a miss), going to talk about fingering. There is no way, no matter how embarrassing it is to write about, that I can pen a chapter on hands without writing about it. Wine, anyone?

Even the word is problematic. In fact, I wouldn't be surprised if kidz today call it something else – probably something completely random like 'badgering', or 'cheeseboarding' (God, I am so middle class), or 'Mexican-waving'. I'm not sure I can face asking the eighteen-year-old babysitter. She may quit. Even the internet doesn't know. And yes, I am about to clear my search history.

In my life I have had some bad fingering times and I have had some good fingering times. One experience that left quite an impression was during a cinema date. One particular boyfriend, uniquely, knew his way around a woman like a concert pianist knows his way around a piece of Wagner, and showed me how much more fun the cinema can be if you take your pants off. I have no idea what the film was about, or even what the film was. All I know was that I was grateful it was a quiet night and not many people wanted to see that particular film. But that night is now etched into my memory in vivid Technicolor as one of the hottest dates I have ever been on.

I really don't want to do this but I have to talk about the bad, or less sensational experiences. For me, as for many girls, this is the first eyebrow-raising physical experience you have with a boy. At that time in my life, when hormones were beginning to run riot around my being, I wasn't too discerning; I was just happy to have some attention and hoped The Boy wouldn't notice I had absolutely *no* idea what I was doing, what was going to happen or how I was expected to react. So I was, essentially, like a passive sack of potatoes (as opposed to an active sack of potatoes). A happy sack of potatoes, I must add. However, whilst not being mind-blowing, on the whole these experiences were explorative and fun.

And they went a little like this:

- get invite to party
- say yes to party
- buy crushed velvet jacket and tartan trousers from Kookai
- curl hair with mother's curling iron
- put on ice-white lipstick
- steal brother's cigarettes
- go to party
- drink as much Archers and lemonade as possible
- dance to 2 Unlimited
- be approached by boy
- be snogged rabidly by boy
- be taken to sofa by boy
- sit still whilst boy puts his hands down pants
- hope that boy doesn't rip new tights
- sit still whilst boy puts his hands up love tunnel
- say goodbye to boy
- dance to Haddaway
- drink more Archers and lemonade
- laugh with friends
- be collected by a responsible adult
- talk about experience with friends for the next three months
- go to Pizza Hut with parents and pretend that the party was, like, really boring and there was nothing at all of any nature to report

The only time it wasn't fun was when, at a party, one boy was far too enthusiastic and went too far north and sent me jumping about a foot into the air. I think that was when I officially broke my hymen. Not as original as my friend who did it riding a horse but one of 'those' life moments nonetheless.

But, for all of the embarrassment of fingering as a way of learning about biology, most of the time it was all very innocent and didn't in any way feel as grubby as it seems right now as I sit here in a grown-up boho coffee shop with a three-pound latte and nice leather sofas squirming at the memories.

But, before we move on to a less squirmy subject, I'd also like to give a moment to the role fingers play in foreplay. Fingers are not just useful when you are starting to engage in sexual activity but are something to be enjoyed at all stages of sexual life. A little like playing the piano, it's something that can be rushed over or relished and done with skill. Fingering, and I can only speak from a woman's perspective here, is an important part of foreplay and often can be the main event. Some of my experiences have led me to believe that it is considered to be a little like turning the oven on and is thus tackled in the same way as trying to get a stain out of a cushion. However, some of my experiences have also led me to believe that it is not something to be overlooked. I know I am talking in annoying vague euphemisms so here it is bluntly. Fingering can feel amazing. It's something to read up on. It can be a winner for everyone.

So, in conclusion, fingering can be bad, it can be good and it can be unbelievable, but, without a doubt, it is a horrible, ungraceful term for something that is, mostly, pretty fun and pretty hot.

## Masturbation

You are more than welcome to read this section of the book through your fingers (another excellent use for them) as this is also a little bit of a touchy subject, so to speak. It shouldn't really be. And, thanks to Caitlin Moran, the Goddess of Masturbation (I hope she relishes that and doesn't want to hunt me down and beat me with a rabbit), I have been inspired to think and talk as openly about this as I possibly can. Caitlin has shared more about the realities of wanking than any other woman. And I'm not talking about the sensual 'touching myself' type of masturbating, i.e. the kind that you might find on a porn site, the point of which is entirely to titillate the viewer (though of course there is nothing wrong with a spot of titillation – good Skype sex often begins with extremely pretty but very impractical, often uncomfortable, underwear and the unspoken potential of all parties putting their hands down their pants).

No, I'm talking about the very delicious, wonderful, utterly normal lady-wanking for the lady's sake and for only the sake of the lady. This is being done, and has been done, by most female people across the globe since the moment women realized that they had fingers, which I reckon was pretty much straight away.

There are a few things, apart from logistics and hand cramp, which hinder the joy of wanking for woman:

## The Myth

The first is the myth that women don't have a high sex drive, and the subsequent shame felt when girls grow up and realize that they do love (good) sex and that masturbating feels amazing, is free and is much less calorific than eating cake. So, having realized at the tender age of sixteen (quite a slow realization considering my early encounter with the shower head) that orgasms were extremely great and since being at a girls' boarding school sex was not easily on tap, I admitted to myself that I probably wanted to masturbate every day. Twice if I had the opportunity. Three times if it was a Saturday and I didn't have netball.

But the problem was I felt such shame, and thus the thing that I wanted to do became something I didn't want to do, but did anyway because of being a human, and then dealt with the guilt that followed. Which was all extremely unnecessary. I looked around for any sign that another girl or woman, even if it was just one, might possibly also be enjoying the delights of 'me time' and found that, in fact, the evidence showed that I was very much alone. No Disney princess takes herself off for a quickie in the woods, no other girl at my school ever admitted to nipping off to the stationery cupboard, no female heroine in any movie ever put her hand down her pants, even to adjust a wedgie (Wonder Woman must have – those Spandex pants were ripe for riding up her bottom), and no telly character that I've ever encountered is late for work because she just fancied a triple-whammy (one of the many perks of being a woman).

## The Silence

Most girls grow up with silence surrounding this subject. Real actual women (well, girls that I was at school with) never talked about it. So the message that I got, loud and clear, was that women do not and should not wank, or even want to wank, and I was well weird for wanting to and doing it and then doing it again sometimes quite quickly afterwards. Boys grow up with masturbation jokes, they swap magazines, they share stories, they tease each other with ease – it is just an accepted part of their early sexual life and an expected part of learning about their bodies. Only a few days ago I was with a guy who joked that the housekeeping staff of the hotel he was staying in were sick of his enthusiastic use of tissues and had protested by leaving the tissue box on his pillow. He told me this anecdote without blinking. I can safely say that if this had happened to most women, they would be mortified (of course this actual situation wouldn't have happened to a woman as biologically we are wonderfully neat and contained in this department); they certainly wouldn't bring it up as a funny story to tell to a group of colleagues.

## Long Nails

I know it's a bit of a curveball but let's address really, really long nails, as they are most definitely an obstacle for 'playing a piano solo'. Perhaps it's just my experience of them, but long nails aren't that fun – I tried them once for a BBC Three documentary (*Cherry's Cash Dilemmas*) and remember standing in my hotel room at the end of a very long night wondering how the bloody Nora I was meant to undo my jeans/make a cup of tea/brush my teeth. In the end, after trying a safety pin, a bottle opener and the corner of the radiator (all involving what I believe to be advanced yoga moves) I had to call the director in to help me de-robe. Now I'm all for the freedom to adorn ourselves however we wish but when you can't take your own trousers off it's probably time to reassess.

That said, this is the woman who is writing this whilst wearing a pair of pants that don't quite cover the fullness of her butt cheeks and therefore keep riding up my bottom, making me a bit squirmy and uncomfortable but, right now, it's worth it because they are really pretty. So if they make you feel lovely, Long Live Long Nails. But never try to masturbate whilst wearing them. Ouch.

## Fantasy Wanking

What's so crazy is that women are built so perfectly, beautifully, wonderfully for masturbation. There are so many ways, so many variations, to how we are turned on and how we orgasm. And we are so neatly contained. We don't start off with a giant totem pole giving our intentions away and, during it, we can be as subtle and covert as someone simply rearranging their pants – think about how obvious and energetic a guy has to be – and at the end of it we generally don't need a tissue.

But masturbation for personal lady satisfaction (so nothing like we see in porn or *Nuts* or anywhere in the media at all) is actually not very sexy to the observer and is often referred to as . . . well, nothing, as we generally don't feel safe to ever mention it. And this type of wanking looks like nothing much other than a woman with her hands under the duvet and a fixed expression on the ceiling or closed eyes depending on how tired she is/what's on telly/how long she has been going (it sometimes take bloody ages – especially if you're simultaneously half watching *Game of Thrones*).

Women do not – I feel pretty confident in saying – put on lacy underwear before they do it. We do it whilst we're still in our favourite very tatty tracksuit bottoms that should have gone in the wash a week ago but it's too painful not to have them even for twenty-four hours. Yes, we 'touch ourselves' in our old, holey, Crunchy Nut cornflakes-stained pyjamas and big comfy pants that cup our whole entire butt cheek, as nature intended. We also do not – again a generalization but still feeling confident – arch our backs and stroke our décolletage (great word) and play with our nipples whilst sucking our index finger. Firstly, if we were to do that it would be tricky to get on with the task in hand and secondly it's wasted energy and I, for one, am far too focused on visualizing some excellently hot scenario (not feeling quite brave enough to expand on that can of worms – although I promise it does not involve any cans or any worms of any description). So in porn the wanking women writhe about in back-arching ecstasy but in reality we don't. Why would we? We are fully engaged in something absolutely delicious, that is just for us. We don't care what we look like; we care how it feels – other than the hot fantasy in our minds, the only other thought is how long before we have to get up and go to work.

It's a bit like one of my favourite meals: sexfast. Stay with me, this is a tangent but it all comes good . . . Sexfast is the meal between supper and breakfast and, for me, it happens any time between 1 and 4 a.m., either after dancing in a club for hours or after lots of sex. It involves standing at the fridge like an angry bear, mindlessly shoving your pie hole with whatever your rabid hands can grab (usually a combination of old salami, processed cheese and a slice of stale birthday cake). And, because you are satiating a hunger like no other, it tastes better than anything you've ever had in even the smartest of establishments. And, like masturbation (thank you for staying with me, here is the link, I promise), to really delight in its deliciousness it must be done without any self-consciousness and therefore it is best done alone.

So there is Real Wanking and then there is Porn Wanking. I've watched the latter and really, really asked myself whether I'm missing something. I want to be sexually open-minded but I can't deny that, to me, the girls just don't look like they're having a good time. The look in their eyes is the same as when I'm whisking eggs to make a meringue. Neither happy nor unhappy, but definitely not in a sexy place. Just, like, doing something. And I think that the portrayal of women masturbating in porn, which was the first and only time I've ever encountered other women masturbating, con- tributed to me feeling that what actually happens is not, well, what a woman's meant to do. They also often only touch themselves for a few seconds and I take consider- ably longer to reach the boil.

But even now at the age of thirty-four, and knowing fully that masturbating does not make you go blind and that most women do it and that doing it every day or using toys does not make you a sex fiend or send you straight to hell, I'm still very nervous/not going to bring it up in conversation with even my closest friends. But this vexes me because I am so very curious. Just imagine, right now, how many women are gleefully getting on with a good session of private time in private? Lots and lots. But how many of those will feel shame or never speak of it or worry that they are a little bit pervy?

Joyfully the solution is in all of our hands. We can just take a leaf out of the boys' book and laugh about it, talk about it, tease each other and gradually break the illusion that women don't do it. So I am going to set myself a challenge this week and try to broach the conversation with other women. (OK, I'm going to start on the nursery slopes and talk to my close friends as opposed to random strangers in the supermarket queue.) And, of course, I would love you to have a go as well. And I will let you know how it goes, but only if you do too.

## Writing

The other magic thing hands can do is write. Glorious, glorious writing. This has been one of the great constants and sources of sanity in my life. If I'm dealing with a particularly tricky situation and my thoughts dart around like a wild deer trapped in a Fiat Punto on a hot day, the act of writing forces them to behave in a linear way and makes everything slow down.

I started my first diary when I was nine and the entry was an exciting 'I had a sleepover with Antonia today and school was poo and my brother is being annoying.' I can't really explain the inclination, but from then on, up until I started making immersive documentaries, I kept diaries. At the start it was just a record of my fascinating daily activities, such as the titillating: 'Hung out with Lucy and Antonia today, we had some strawberry laces, then we watched *Byker Grove*, then I went home and Mum made shepherd's pie and then I went to bed.' Thankfully (ish) they progressed on to love angst (boys, boys, boys), philosophizing (who/what/how am I?) and self-esteem (am I too fat/not pretty enough/not clever enough). I know it's now hard to believe, having bared my soul in television documentaries aired to the nation, but I really *did* write the diaries without the slightest intention of ever showing them to another living soul. And whilst they were never a secret, lots of my good friends didn't even know I kept diaries.

The result is that they are very, very raw. For a long time I never read them – they were just stacked up at the back of my cupboard and forgotten about. But later, on the rare occasion I did read them, I tried to view them through the eyes of a loving older sister. Because, often, the content is fairly unlovable. I really did not mince my words and I was sometimes a gigantic bitch, or a painfully pained teenager, or a cringingly righteous twenty-something. You name it, I've ticked that stereotype. But when I reread them, I do try to understand that I was doing the best that I could at the time with the information that I had at the time. And, whilst we're here, I think that's deeply informed how I view people – sometimes it's easy to be perplexed or to judge other people's decisions, but we are all just doing our *best* with the *best* information we have at the time. And that's all we can do. Nothing more.

OK, back to being a cringeworthy teenager and on to the subject of love letters. Whilst I love my MacBook like I love my children, I do feel the loss of letters. Handwritten, textured, Tippexed letters. At boarding school I remember the elated excitement of pelting down the stairs in the morning and gathering round the post table like sweaty commuters circling the last seat. I was always surprised that no one did themselves or other girls serious injury as they desperately searched for their own names on the mysterious envelopes. And sometimes, oh lo and behold, joy of joys, there it was, ready to be torn open and read and reread and passed around the class and the dormitory and back again until it looked like an ancient scroll from biblical times – an actual letter. All for me. Magic. Mostly it was from my mum and dad (I wish I had kept those), but very occasionally it was from a real human boy. And this was treated like treasure from the tombs of the Egyptian pyramids.

Now, nearly two decades later, knee-deep in the world of tap-tap-tapping and Googling and swiping and ctrl-alt-deleting, I can say that no email, no matter how beautiful or poetic or full of love or feeling, comes close to the intimacy and excitement of a handwritten letter. There is something deeply personal about it. There is so much more to read than the words – the choice of paper, the handwriting, the smell. (I remember spraying CK One on to one of my most cringeworthy efforts whilst also listening to Take That's 'I Want You Back' so that I could emote on to the page with even *more* intensity).

A letter is tactile; you can hold it in your hands, smell it, store it, and reread it again and again. A letter is less clinical than an email and, because of the inability of the writer to delete their words very easily once committed to paper, there is a wonderful authenticity and spontaneity. The boy's hand has actually touched it – oh God, when I think of the potency of that image for me as a male-starved boarding-school girl! You can imagine them sitting, thinking, composing, taking the time out of their busy schedule (of eating toast) to pen a real-life love letter to you. All for you. Not cut 'n' paste, but thoughts and feelings that give you your first exciting experience of being seen and loved by someone other than your mum or your pet dog. They've not only taken the effort to pen their emotions but have made a practical effort – they've found somewhere quiet, bought stationery, a pen, a stamp and walked down to the postbox to send it. It's uniquely flattering.

And that's perhaps the nugget of why I find hands so beautiful. They are such an honest and hard-to-hide indicator of how we are feeling: the steady, confident hand of a surgeon, the fingers that pick nervously as a student waits for the exam papers to be turned over, the desperate palms clasped together of someone willing a letter to arrive. Whether they are adorned with trendy chunky brushed-gold rings or powerful statement diamonds, or henna or tattoos or have short bitten nails or long painted talons, hands communicate like no other part of the body. They are magic.

# 3. Letter to My Brain: Education, Money, Work, Brain Food

*Greetings and salutations, Brain,*

*There aren't many parts of my body that I wish were bigger but if you wanted to increase in size I would not complain one little bit. Well, hang tight, I don't wish you were physically bigger as then none of my hats would fit, but I wouldn't mind if you had a bigger capacity for things like names (then I could walk down the street without having to dive into shops to avoid any awkwardness), trivial information (then I could take part in pub quizzes without getting clammy) and people's birthdays (I'm sorry to all my friends and family – the information just seems to go in one ear and then fall out of my bottom).*

*I would like to say thank you for those fifteen years of school – no one likes exams, and regurgitating information for three hours in a silent room is most definitely not your happy place, but you did it. Considering your natural strengths are extracurricular, I'm grateful that somehow you wangled your way through the school system and emerged the other end without imploding and with some confidence intact.*

*However, for all your wonderful resilience, I do have a bone to pick with you. You're good at many things and we've got this far without a prison sentence or falling down a mine shaft, but you do occasionally let me down. It sometimes feels as though you're not on my side – is that fair? It's as though there is something deep within you that's wired to tell me I'm not good enough. Whether it's the way that I look, the way that I parent, my worth in the workplace, comparing myself to other women – your neural pathways seem set on self-sabotage. You can be my worst enemy.*

*But as I get older I see that, because you are not a fixed entity, it's important to control you rather than be controlled by you. Like a wild horse, you are powerful and either I harness that or run the risk of being kicked in the face. I know that if I feed you good things, you produce good results and if I feed you crap then, well, we know where that goes. So I apologize for all the rubbish I've been ingesting – I'm older and wiser and so I will try to give you more nutritious, affirming, broadening information. But if I do stray and end up reading an article about someone's bottom or love life or cellulite, let's maybe work together to put it in the 'Delete' folder, yes? Go, team.*

## Education

The first time I fell out with my brain was in 1989 during a maths lesson at primary school. My teacher was a huge, buxom, rosy-cheeked woman who could have been Mrs Santa Claus had she not been so bad tempered. Sadly, because my encounter with this maths teacher was so horrible, I'll never know whether I'm genetically bad at maths or whether it's because I was repeatedly told I was bad at maths. And I can't help but think, because it was the girls she picked on, even though she herself was female, that she just didn't think maths was for girls. I wonder if she felt we should all be focusing on making cheese twists in home economics or painting pictures of kittens in funny hats (to prepare us for the grown-up world of office Instagram-offs). There's plenty of evidence that girls – and boys – still tend to be socialized in subtle and not so subtle ways to see science, maths and technology subjects as 'for boys'. As the wonderful Cordelia Fine puts so pithily in her book *Delusions of Gender*, 'Boys do not pursue mathematical activities at a higher rate than girls do because they are better at mathematics. They do so, at least partially, because they think they are better.'

This particular teacher had perhaps had some bad career advice and didn't seem to like children or teaching. I think she would have been much happier being a butcher, a baker or a candlestick-maker. Anything, in fact, other than a teacher. But as a result of the bad career advice, she had a bit of a temper and if she asked a question and the reply wasn't instant, she would throw chalk (yes, I was educated back in the Stone Age) or a wooden blackboard wiper or anything else she had to hand. And she was unfortunately quite a good shot and would often get us right in the kisser.

On one particular day when, paralysed by fear, I hesitated to answer a question, she pulled me to the front of the class and shouted: '*YOU NEED TO PULL YOUR*

*SOCKS UP, YOUNG LADY!'* and, because I was nine and had never heard this expression before, I pulled my socks up. She exploded. I think every drop of blood in my body drained through my feet and into the floorboards and I turned a shade of grey that Farrow & Ball would probably call 'Shitting Oneself'. She then sent me outside for the rest of the class, where I wondered if it was possible to die from heart palpitations and sweaty palms (yes, I think it probably is). Over the next few months this happened a few more times in different flavours of awful until one day I decided it was probably a good idea to stop talking altogether as then she might leave me alone or forget I existed.

So, throughout the day and then afterwards, when my mum collected me from school, I would be silent. Which, when you are nine, seems like a genius plan but is obviously very scary for a mum used to having a chatterbox bounce into the car and scoff a chocolate flapjack whilst banging on about Take That. And it gradually became so bad that I would hide under the glove compartment in a little ball. It seemed like a foolproof plan at the time to make myself invisible.

And this is when my mum became Tiger Beast Fire-Eating Person-Biting Lady. Normally the sweetest, kindest, most gentle five-foot-four woman you could meet, with a bob so neat and brushed it merely vibrates in the wind, she morphed into a tweed-clad ninja before my eyes. I remember with absolute crystal vividness sitting in the cloakroom with my best friend Lucy Austin, looking through the thin pane of glass into the classroom whilst my mum gave this teacher a piece of her mind. Even though the teacher was a good two feet taller than my mum, she looked terrified. My mum has a way with words and never once did she need to raise her voice – her eyes said it all – although at one point she *did* allow herself a desk slam. I didn't know whether this was about to make my life better or worse but I made a mental note never to mess with my mum.

Thankfully my life at school dramatically improved after that and the teacher never so much as looked my way again, which meant I could end my vow of silence, much to the sadness of my friends who were probably enjoying some peace. Happy days. But sadly she did have a lasting effect and more than two decades later, faced with any kind of numerical question, my brain turns into jam and I have a complete brain-freeze. And whilst I've tried various methods to change this, it's something I haven't yet been able to rewire. And in a world that revolves around money, and now as a freelancer in charge of my own tax and income and trying to understand mortgage repayment rates and VAT, it's extremely inconvenient to struggle with numbers. Which is why I am now so conscious of the profound effect teachers can have on children.

It was in sixth form that I encountered the particularly glorious Mrs Rowell, my history of art teacher. She was elegant and cultured, with a beautiful Czech accent and her grey hair always in a chic up-do. She would tell stories that captivated us all – about the artist's life, about what life was like in ye olden days and why the paintings blew people away and changed history. I thought she was the best thing since Bovril.

I started her class when I was sixteen and had been struggling with my grades. I was incredibly frustrated because, unlike a lot of my friends who seemed to get away with doing almost nothing and still come out shining, I actually read the books and did the work. But I still came out with average-to-low grades with slightly more polite versions of comments such as 'What on earth are you talking about?' and 'Please be less crap'. One day Mrs Rowell asked me to come to her office after school. And this is where she told me that, after reading a handful of my essays, she had an idea of why I wasn't nailing them. She noticed that all the information was there, but it was just a giant splurge of thoughts. And, within a few meetings, she taught me how to create a piece of work with a clear beginning, middle and end. Observing how my brain worked, she suggested I read the textbooks first, without trying to half write random paragraphs in an over-excited way only to find that they didn't relate to each other. She also told me to write the conclusion *first*. And it worked like a charm. In the space of one month, this wonderful woman took me from a struggling student to an A student. Just because she had taken the time to observe and understand. I went from feeling like a bit of a thickie to someone whose confidence academically grew exponentially. I even started using words like 'exponentially'. And because all of my subjects were essay-based, I applied the same method to everything I did and my entire school experience was transformed. And here I am two decades later applying the same techniques to this book. Without Mrs Rowell this whole book would be a blithering mess/ not exist. This is the power of one teacher caring. Without a doubt she changed my life. Teachers can be life-changing; we should pay them more. Amen.

I do feel lucky that my secondary-school experience was mostly amazing. I loved my friends, I loved sport (I spent fifty per cent of the time falling into the stereotype of the public-school girl by carrying a hockey or lacrosse stick around like a third limb) and I loved boarding. It was like a sleepover every night because it *was* a sleepover every night. It taught me some incredibly useful things – how to negotiate female power politics, how to make a three-course meal using only a kettle and, most importantly, how to pick my battles. Because if you're a bit of a cow one day, you have to wake up next to the person who you were a bit of a cow to. You then have to have breakfast with that person and walk to school with them. And then have supper with them and brush your teeth next to them and so on and so on. So, generally, it was best to be a cow as little as possible.

I also learned that the saying 'Never let the sun go down on an argument' was utter cods-crap. *Always* let the sun go down on an argument because, ninety per cent of the time, you wake up not really caring about it any more. Or if you do still care about it, you're in a better frame of mind to talk about it. We did of course have some blazing arguments but they were fairly quickly forgotten once we realized it was TV night (Thursday) or doughnut day (Thursday). Thursdays are still my favourite day of the week.

Whilst I had no problem with being at an all-girls school, I do think there are *some* problems with same-sex education. In the real world, where people eat doughnuts on days other than Thursdays, women and men interact together. So, why not start learning how to do that from when we're young, in the care of teachers who can guide us?

They say that school days are the happiest of your life but I'm extremely thankful that, for me, that didn't play out. Even though my school experience was good, I much prefer *not* being at school – I like being able to eat Crunchy Nut cornflakes at 2 a.m., I like wearing what I want, I like going to bed when I want and earning money for work I've done rather than gold stars. Actually that's a lie – I really miss the gold stars. I wish someone had told me (they probably did, many times) that the reason it's a good idea to work hard at school is because then you're much more likely to have a cool job afterwards. And having a job you like and, perhaps *love*, is worth *every* minute in the library, *every* second of cramp in your hand from writing (or typing, because it's not 1950) and *every* late-night cramming session, prising your bloodshot eyes open with All-Bran – *it's all worth it.* They should emblazon that on every wall in every school in the world (minus the All-Bran bit).

## *Money – or the Pay-Gap Puzzle*

The 9<sup>th</sup> of November has recently become a significant date for women but sadly not one to celebrate. This is when women go to work for free. Yes, this is when we get up early, brush our teeth, frog-jump our way into some tights, pack our lunches, brave the wind and rain, get our face stuck in someone's armpit on a crowded train, input data, care for patients, mark homework, forecast finances, bake bread, stack shelves, all for free. Freeeeee! No money! Gratis! Sweet F to the A. Whilst a dude is paid actual money that can be spent on things like food and heat and water and socks. So useful.

With the pay gap still at a whopping 19.1 per cent (including part-time), things have changed little in the past few years, even though the conversation has been getting louder. I was surprised by a friend's comment recently as they struggled to understand why there was such a hullabaloo about this, as things have clearly improved significantly in the four decades since women first protested about pay inequality. I then suggested he work for free for the final two months of the year, in solidarity with women, and he said no thanks and that he understood my point. The women of Denmark win the prize for highlighting the issue in a wonderfully slick and efficient way. Their unions urge female members to go on strike from the 9th November until the end of December, thus eradicating the pay gap in one swift move. Clever.

So. What I don't understand is how it is that girls start off doing better than boys at school, and then, fast-forward ten years, boys are doing better in the workplace and rising up the food chain faster and with better pay? I know it sounds like a generalization but this is well researched and generally accepted and I Googled it so it must be true. It doesn't make sense. What happens in those ten years up to the point when boys overtake girls, at exactly the moment that work starts to be rewarded with actual *real* money rather than stickers and a smiley face?

Why, oh why, in 2016, is this still happening?

I have a few theories.

1. Girls pick up the message that their competitive urges should be channelled into winning the attention of men rather than success at work.
2. Girls don't feel comfortable talking about money and our sense of self-worth in the workplace doesn't match a man's, almost like we're not completely sure we belong there yet.
3. Women go off and have babies. Dicks.

On the first point, is it just me or when girls are described as 'ambitious' does it sometimes sound like a subtle insult? It's somehow inferred that they aren't a real woman, that they are aggressive and unpleasant, that perhaps they might even have fangs and furry palms and smell like washing after it's been left in the machine for too long.

Why can't a woman be competitive at work and also be entirely feminine? I am competitive but it doesn't mean I am cut-throat or without morals or work ethics or want to watch anyone in pain as I trample all over them whilst wearing running spikes. I will work as hard as I can and hope that I win the job, but if I don't win I don't throw my toys out of the pram or pull anyone's hair or claw their face (just that one time). As that glorious broad Bette Davis said, 'When a man gives his opinion, he's a man. When a woman gives her opinion, she's a bitch.'

Why can't a girl have a healthy, balanced sense of competition, just as a man can? Well, the answer is of course she can. Working hard and wanting to win are not incongruous with anything that a woman is. However, there *is* something in our mass media that contradicts this. And because my daughter is six and I read to her every night, I can't help but scrutinize the books available and the messages they send to her at such a formative age when she is absorbing everything like a sponge.

I used to love the idea of my daughter and me being tucked up cosy in bed whilst I read her the Disney fairy tales that I loved growing up. But, as an adult, I look at these stories in a new light. The female characters are, well, a bit lame. They flounce around in impractical dresses, with borderline malnutrition, going against the good advice given to them, getting into trouble, crying in the woods and sitting about waiting to be saved by someone really dishy. They're beautiful but they're totally incompetent. They're hailed as heroines, the ideal woman, with their thin necks, small waists, long locks, stunning attire and little shiny shoes. Yet, as an adult, if I was faced with one I'd probably shake her and send her on a military survival course pronto to learn how to turn her wee into drinking water and how to tie her hair back at the first sign of trouble (see Exhibit A: Ripley in *Aliens* – when the shit hits the proverbial fan the first thing she does is reach for a hairband, because if you try fighting a gigantic slimy ant with your hair blowing in your face you are definitely going to get pronged by a horrible weird impregnator probe that comes out of its mouth).

Whilst in some ways these fairy stories are as innocent as vanilla ice cream, what message are these heroines giving our little girls at such an influential age? Which women are they reading about, pretending to be, fantasizing about, dressing up as? Utter lame-os, that's who. Where are the female characters who make shit happen? Who climb to the top of the metaphorical mountain? Who solve puzzles and win competitions and lose gracefully whilst working out how to do it better next time? Well, thankfully there are *some* fantastic books that contain ace mega-babes of excellence. And this is joyfully happening more and more in print, film and television.

Some absolute crackers:

- *You Can't Scare A Princess!* – Gillian Rogerson and Sarah McIntyre
- *The Paper Bag Princess* – Robert Munsch and Michael Martchenko
- *Matilda* – Roald Dahl
- Anything with Dora the Explorer
- *Princess Smartypants* – Babette Cole

(And, while we're on the subject, my own feminist book list is:

- *How To Be a Woman* – Caitlin Moran
- *Fat Is a Feminist Issue* – Susie Orbach
- *Lean In* – Sheryl Sandberg
- *We Should All Be Feminists* – Chimamanda Ngozi Adichie
- *A Book for Her* – Bridget Christie
- *Everyday Sexism* – Laura Bates
- *Not That Kind of Girl* – Lena Dunham

But, for little girls, the Disney mafia is still the prominent force and, whilst I would love to ban them at home, when all the other children in the class are debating their favourite princess, it feels too mean to exclude my daughter from this fun. So I *do* read my daughter these books (whilst sneakily changing the words to make the main character seem less of a feckless plonker) and just hope that she will see enough women in her life who *will* chase the metaphorical ball to understand that it's OK to be competitive and have boobs and be an excellent, lovely person.

So much for girls learning at a young age that they shouldn't be seen to be competitive or go-getting.

Also, I wonder whether women don't feel comfortable talking about money because we're not completely, a hundred per cent, through and through sure we belong or are welcome in the workplace. I have always gone into a new job with a feeling of wanting to impart my great thanks to whoever is hiring me. In fact, my idea of a successful meeting goes something like this: 'Hi there, thank you so much for taking me on! Thank you for letting me in the building! Can I give YOU some money to let me do the work? Thank you for your time! What a great meeting! Goodbye!'

I don't think I have ever, or would ever, ask how much someone is going to pay me. Good. God. No. Other than the documentary I made *about* money, I don't think I've ever said the word 'money' in a meeting. Yet my fear of talking about money is crackers. It's *my job* to have tricky conversations about taboo subjects. Why is it that I'm happy to ask someone about how they lost their virginity but I won't ask my employer about how much money I'm going to be paid? In fact, only last week I had a meeting with a newspaper to discuss writing an article for them.

And because I was in the middle of writing this chapter, I decided I needed to put my money where my mouth was and bring up the subject of how much I was going to be paid. So, bracing myself and with a pained expression, I asked if they (the commissioner and my agent) had talked '*numbers*'?

But this was my *best* shot. I couldn't even bring myself to say the actual word 'money'. And I felt so embarrassed to even be asking. As I walked home through Soho, which was buzzing with women doing all sorts of cool, fun jobs, I wondered, *Is it just me?* How do other women learn to talk about money directly? How many other women struggle with this? How on earth are we going to close the pay gap if we/I can't even ask the simple question of how much I'm going to be paid? Is it that I'm scared of being perceived to be greedy? And if so, why don't men fear this? Why is the dynamic that Men + Work = Reward whereas Women + Work = Grateful?

My good friend runs a medium-sized company of about thirty-five staff and, after a decade of carrying out staff appraisals, he has observed that men and women behave very differently when it comes to asking for a pay rise. Men, in general, come into the meeting with a sense of confidence, wanting to talk about how their skill and talent has increased the company's profits and how their pay rise should therefore reflect this. And then they negotiate hard until they have the best possible deal. Women, on the other hand, tend to bring a sense of gratitude, and often accept the first offer they are given. And in that moment the difference may only be small, perhaps two or three per cent, but over time this accumulates and we end up with a significant pay gap and feeling a bit miffed. In his words: 'I'm surprised the pay gap isn't bigger, really.'

Looking at this, it does seem that self-worth is the root of the problem. I, and many other women I know, struggle to fully embrace the monetary value they bring to a job and to convince someone that my skills deserve to be rewarded with dollar dollar bill ya'll (or sterling). And I wonder whether this is because there is something deep within me, deep within my brain, that's not entirely sure I belong in the work world and that any minute now someone could tap me on the shoulder and tell me to put my apron back on and crack on with making them a chicken pie already.

So much has changed for women in the last couple of generations. Back in the 1970s, it was still very much the norm for mums to stay at home, yet now sixty-seven per cent of British women aged sixteen to sixty-four are in work, which is astonishingly high given that this will include mothers who have just given birth, as well as those unable to work because of illness, disability or because they are caring for others (still a predominantly female thing). In fact, the gap between the number of men and women who hold a job is narrowing year by year; the percentage of men who work is down from ninety-two per cent in 1971 to seventy-six per cent today. The way the trends are going, these figures will be equal soon. It's a monumental change in just a few decades.

When I was at school, only a couple of my friends' mothers worked, and now *every single one* of my female friends works, or is preparing to go back to work after having a baby. That is a gigantic shift to take place in just a couple of generations. We've gone from nought to sixty in five seconds.

And so, is it any wonder that women aren't completely sure of their place in the work world? That we are looking over our shoulder at the women before us, women like my mum, who weren't encouraged to find a career but rather felt their place was at home, and whilst we have a sense of glee and thankfulness that our options have opened up, I wonder if we don't entirely trust it. Yet.

I imagine, I hope, that our daughters won't have this insecurity. I think that time will do its magical thing and they will see their mums and aunts and godmothers working and they will start to think about *what* their careers might be, rather than if they *can* have a career. They will grow up in a world where this isn't even in question. Of course, they may want to be stay-at-home mums, but rather than feeling that's where they *should* be, they will be able to choose freely.

Keen to set my daughter's imagination running wild with career dreams, and so I can start living vicariously through her – as we all know is very healthy (ahem) – we often talk about what she'd like to do when she grows up. And I love that the answer changes all the time and I'm immediately aglow with premature pride as I imagine her doing something that makes her very happy.

But let's face it, it's not always easy for women once they get to the stage of juggling a career and motherhood, even if they have managed to land their dream job. I remember the moment *I* caved from the pressure of it all. I was in the middle of making a documentary on parenting when I realized that I wasn't coping with juggling parenting and work. Oh the irony. Because of the nature of my work, I can't always be sure of what day I will be away filming. And because, at the time, we were in a one-bedroom flat and I hadn't yet got my head around nurseries (you do slightly need a PhD in childcare to understand the options), we had a day nanny. She would charge £80 for a day running from eight till six. This is standard. But my hours are totally unpredictable as filming ends when filming ends so sometimes when I was meant to be home at 6 p.m. and, due to cancellations or a location pulling out or a dog barking or a vehicle reversing and having to wait for the sound to clear, I would be back three or four hours late. And that would be an extra £40 and a huge dollop of 'sorry sorry sorry' to the angry nanny who had evening plans. I did this dance for a year, spending every penny I earned booking childcare for five days a week when I was only really using three, and spending most evenings and mornings either begging for favours or apologizing. It was horrible.

So what to do? Well, cheaper childcare would be a good place to start. I'm not sure why the government hasn't caught up with this – there is a huge generation of working, voting women who are being checkmated when going back into their careers. How do we live in a country where you can claim for a chauffeur but not a nanny? How is childcare more expensive than an average mortgage? How, if you have two or three sprogs, are you meant to even dream of going back to work?

I have no answers on this one sadly. Just frustrations and a desire for childcare to be affordable and for women to be able to choose to return to work without tearing their hair out at the choice of either working for free or staying at home and missing out on a job they adore and watching a career they have worked hard to build slip away from them. Yeah. No biggie.

So there are many reasons why the pay gap hasn't closed. Leaving the workplace for large chunks of time on maternity leave, a lack in confidence and unaffordable childcare are all contributing factors. But thankfully all of these can be changed. By both parents deciding on how they want to share maternity leave and more jobs being done from home or on flexible time, with more government help with childcare vouchers and the ever-changing perspective on what it means to be a woman, I hope that we'll soon be able to celebrate the 9th of November for a good reason.

## Women Being in Control of Their Money

And so, in the same way that I believe our daughters will grow up without any doubt that they belong in the workplace, I believe that our daughters will see us managing our own money and will have no hesitation when talking about or handling their finances. And this is possibly one of the most important things I'd like my daughter to grasp. It's one of the biggest frustrations about my education, and I think it's one of the most dangerous things for a woman – well, anyone – to overlook: being in control of and on top of your money. Because if you are not on top of things and the poo hits the fan, there are some seriously un-fun consequences. No matter how bad the poo is, or how much has hit the fan, the world keeps spinning and the bills keep coming. And if life does throw poo at you and your fan, at the very least you need to know that there is enough money in the bank, ideally, to see you through whilst you clean the poo from the fan. (That is the end of the fan and poo metaphor, I promise.)

At school I learned many things. I learned how to make a clay ashtray. I learned how to make cheese straws. I learned how to eat an entire marmalade sandwich in an English lesson without getting caught. But somehow I didn't learn how to manage my money. Of course, at eighteen years old my money situation was about £40 (a king's sum in 1999) and so perhaps any income–expenditure information would have gone in one ear and then dissolved instantly. But now I'm thirty-four I see the absolute, unquestionable importance of a woman understanding her finances. There seems to be a hangover of the traditional dynamic where the man brings in and manages the money. I'm not sure how but I fell into that dynamic without even blinking. When I married, it was like something inside of me breathed a huge sigh of relief that I could finally stop worrying about numbers as I'd never had a great relationship with them anyway. Phhhhheeeewwwww.

So gradually I took my eye off the money ball. I focused on making sure the fridge was full of cheese and bread and ham and After Eights (essential) and the house was clean and the children organized and happy and wearing pants and socks. And because I was doing that I could relinquish control. I cringe now when I think about it, but quite recently my eye was so far off the ball that I didn't even know what our monthly outgoings were, what my total annual income was or whether, which is key, our outgoings were being covered by my income. I was the sole breadwinner and yet I had no idea whether I was earning enough to cover our costs. Barking. I just pootled along with my head firmly up my bum. But I told myself that we were a team and that as long as I hadn't misplaced one of the children or forgotten to buy milk, it was a sensible set-up.

It is not a sensible set-up.

It is very, very silly.

Because when everything is all lovely and happy and there are bunnies hopping in the field and the sun is shining and la-di-da then all is fine. But what happens when things aren't OK? I know it sounds cynical but realistically that can and does sometimes happen. And I know too many women who are in such a vulnerable position because if something happened to their boyfriend or husband, they wouldn't know where to start. They don't know which account the mortgage or rent is paid from or how much it is, how much the council tax, water, gas or electricity is. And they have no insurance if their income disappears. And they don't have their own savings pot. Wow. Hard to believe? Well, that was me. I woke up and realized that I had slowly slipped into a very dangerous place. I had become a 1950s housewife without even realizing and something about it felt familiar and comforting.

Something deep within my brain told me that money was the male domain and that contributed to my sense of financial brain-freeze. And this isn't without reason. If I go into the bank with a man, the staff talk to him. They might throw the odd sentence my way but predominately I am not integral to the conversation. If I go for dinner with a man, even if I've produced the plastic, the waiter will hand the pin machine to him. If we get a cab together, the receipt will be handed to him. The list goes on and on. And so, without even *trying* to grasp my finances, I told myself that it was far too complicated and my husband would be better off dealing with it. But that is of course total rubbish.

And so I have spent the past few months (actually, it's more like a year and it's still going on now but it is perhaps slightly less pant-wettingly acute) re-educating myself. Thankfully I found a very unpatronizing accountant who took me through my business finances including the massively entertaining world of Tax and VAT and then I painstakingly went through every single penny coming into my life and going out. It was an incredibly scary but empowering experience. I should have done it years ago. And it was a huge relief to see that it's not rocket science, and I now have a solid(ish) grasp of my finances. Once I had stopped reeling from our family's monthly outgoings (the kids ate dust for a few weeks following that revelation) I was able to make a few changes – switch my phone contracts/electricity provider/stopped using Uber like my personal chauffeur – I made some much needed savings. It was such a relief. And I'm happy to report to those who might feel intimidated by their personal finances that it's much less scary and much less complicated than I thought. And now that I have braved it I feel much more secure.

A shared life is beautiful and an important part of a relationship but when it comes to money I think it's vital that a woman remains as aware of the financial goings-on as the person she shares her life with. Giving up control is just too dangerous and by losing control you lose your freedom.

You lose the freedom to choose if things don't go well, you cap your options and make yourself very vulnerable. And whilst it doesn't sound very romantic, it doesn't change anything about how committed you are to a relationship; in fact, I think by making both parties feel equally empowered and in control and safe it strengthens the bond.

## Money = Taboo

Once you've heard someone discussing, in detail, the challenges their warty bottom presents (an *Embarrassing Bodies* classic), it would be easy to assume that there are no taboo subjects left in the world. But there is one taboo that has remained as tightly locked up as ever before: money. I think most people would rather *pretend* they had a warty bottom than talk about what they earn and, even worse, what they spend.

I'd consider myself to be a fairly open person, but when it comes to money, even outside the workplace, I can feel myself closing off. It's a mixture of embarrassment that I might be earning more/less than the person asking, embarrassment because I don't manage my money well sometimes and embarrassment at how much I spend in Topshop. I'd love to know how much other women spend on clothes and make-up. I have always thought my spending in that area was fairly standard but when I run my eye over my bank statement I can't help wondering whether I have shopping amnesia.

My Lady Family and I share almost everything. We talk about sex and work and health and brain-workings and anxiety and joy and everything in between. But there are a few fields we haven't ploughed. And one of those is money. If my friends asked me how much I earned, it would feel very strange. But I would *love* to know what their finances looked like. Ideally I'd like them to give me an Excel spreadsheet listing how much they spend on clothes, food, cosmetics and fun. Like seeing into someone's handbag or fridge, it would be a fascinating insight into a very private part of them. Other than being a very nosey person, my motive isn't to judge but to use that information as a barometer for how I'm spending.

It's a shame that we're not more open about money. It's hard to learn better practice and to monitor ourselves without hearing about how others are doing it (this is my justification for asking people to hand over their bank statements without them calling the police). And because it's something as important as making sure we've got enough money to pay for the roof over our heads and the food on our tables (and the new trendy felt hat on our heads), perhaps it's time we started sharing more? I wonder why there are so many articles in magazines about what's inside someone's handbag and fridge and wardrobe but I have never seen a single article listing what someone earns and spends. That would be utterly fascinating. Who wants to go first?!

# Money Makes Us Mad

Money can make us behave in bizarre ways. At my most bonkers I would hide shopping bags in the cupboards when I got home, even though I was the breadwinner for our family. I know, very silly. Even though I knew (well, a guess) that we had enough disposable income for me to buy a new pair of slightly shiny green trousers that were, to the naked eye, exactly the same as a pair I already had, I felt guilty for 'wasting' our family money on something I didn't really need. I have now created a watertight justification for why I 'need' the occasional new item, which goes something along the lines of dressing being my creative outlet and creativity is never finished so I shouldn't feel bad for expressing my creativity through new clothes especially if they are slightly shiny and have cute little zips by the ankle. Like, Van Gogh didn't paint *Sunflowers* and put his brush down and proclaim, 'Well, that's that then. I've done art. That's me done. What's next?' Yeah. Like I say, watertight.

My other mad money period was at the start of my third year of university when I was given a credit card. Yes. At the age of twenty-one, with no savings or track record of living within my overdraft, I was *encouraged* by the bank to have a credit card. They might as well have just given me a big stinking stressful debt and cut out the middleman. And, of course, it felt like free money and so that's how I spent it. (I hear that this is about to be remedied and instead of being taught how to iron wax on to cushion covers to make a snazzy pattern, children will learn how to look after their money and not get into a stinking stressful debt – about bloody time.)

It wasn't that I nipped off to Prada or ate at sexy restaurants – I just used it for a travel card (when all my student friends were using the bus), treated my friends to a pub dinner every so often and occasionally indulged in a giant Primark haul. But because nothing was obviously splurgy, it didn't seem like a problem.

At the start I paid off the balance on time and in full, but then after several months of burning my plastic fairly liberally, and it's a bit hazy as to how I let that happen, I found myself with a whopping £3,000 debt. Fuck and fuck. And considering I was earning £5.50 an hour at Starbucks every weekend, that was a *monumental* amount and I knew it would take me three million trillion years to pay it off. So I did what any self-respecting student does and I called my mum. And she did what any self-respecting mum does and told me to create a plan to pay it off. Not quite what I had in mind but now I am deeply, deeply thankful that's how she dealt with it. It was my first experience of debt-fear and it was as cold and icy as a cold and icy shower.

So. I upped my hours at Starbucks, stopped eating out, bought a bicycle and gradually started paying off the debt. Once I had created my plan, it wasn't so bad. It felt like a project and it was certainly less bad than handing over my card at the supermarket checkout and feeling embarrassment and anxiety as I wondered whether it would be declined. My pay-back plan continued after I graduated and through my first job as a marketing assistant and then during my time as a runner at the BBC. I remember sitting in the pub in Shepherds Bush, where all the weary runners gather at the end of a long week, and receiving the text from my bank telling me that I was in the black. It was absolutely, gloriously, wonderfully magic. The feeling that my salary was going into my bank and it was all for me was, well, so relaxing. It wasn't going into the black hole of debt – it was for meeeeeeeeeeee. And so I bought everyone a round and then promised myself to stop doing that.

Even now, if a bank tries to push a credit card on to me (it happens *all* the time), I get cross. I know it's not their fault as it's the company policy but I think it's awful. It's so irresponsible and it's potentially incredibly dangerous for someone. I was lucky in that I didn't have a family at the time and could pootle about on a bike and move back home with my parents if needs be and eat cereal out of a packet for supper without batting an eyelid. But if I were in that situation now, with two children, it would be serious.

Not that full control is for everyone. Back in the day, when the day was 2011, I made a programme about our relationship with money for BBC Three. I met a woman who kept her husband on a tighter leash than her three

Labradors. It was one of the most uncomfortable interviews I have ever done, and not just because of the subject matter. It took place in her dogs' bedroom, which was luxuriously decorated and included a cosy sofa (for her dogs, let's remember), which she sat on. I sat opposite her on the floor, which was, I now know, a huge error. The problem was I didn't realize how bad this seating choice was until we had filmed quite a bit and it was too late to change (continuity). And, as we talked, she watched nonchalantly whilst her three dogs tongued me. (Whilst I think dogs are lovely, it's challenging trying to interview someone whilst they are trying to stick their tongues, three at a time, into your mouth, ear and nose. And she had definitely not been spending their allowance on doggy toothpaste. Yuk.)

During the interview she told me that she felt no guilt at restricting her husband to a £50 a month allowance, even though she didn't work and spent three times that on her dogs. Each week she created a meal plan, which he wasn't allowed to deviate from, and fed him the cheapest, most questionable-looking sausages that definitely contained some kind of animal anus, whilst her dogs dined on steak. Even though he was the breadwinner and she had decided that she couldn't be bothered to work (her words), she didn't let him touch the family finances. I found myself judging like a dirty, dirty judger. I was full to the brim with judgement. I was sure that during my interview with the husband I would hear a story of oppression and bullying. But no. Instead I heard a story of a man who hated any form of responsibility or decision-making. He was completely and utterly complicit. He didn't have to decide where he went, when or what he ate, or worry about a single bill. He was as happy as a hamster. Another beautiful reminder never to judge. Because they were both pleased with the situation. It isn't something that would work for me but it worked perfectly for them. Hearing about how they earned and spent their money, in full detail, was as fascinating as I thought it would be.

For this guy, not being in charge of his own money meant that, yes, he didn't have power or control but it also meant no responsibilities and no worries. For him that was a fair deal.

But for the rest of us who don't relish the idea of handing over all financial control to someone who feeds their dogs fillet steak, I think one of the most important aspects of managing money and regaining control is managing fear. For me, the reason I got into debt was because I stuck my head in the sand. And of course, the problem only got worse. And because I grew up thinking I was bad at maths, I was hugely intimidated by money, so I just ignored it. But I now realize that it's not rocket science. I can do it. And if there is a problem, it's so much better to take a deep breath and look at it head-on. The earlier you do this, the easier the issue is to resolve. Even a few months can make a huge difference. I also found that being accountable to a trusted friend helped me to not stick my head back into the sand. By asking someone to keep a check on how I was doing, I felt less alone and scared and more able to keep on top of it. Yes, money makes the world go round but, really, we are in charge.

## *Work*

I am sometimes asked how I got into presenting and I usually whizz through the past eight years of my life trying to impart enough interesting information without boring the person senseless. I try to take guidance from their closing eyelids and the dribble coming from their mouth as to how many details to include. A bit like showing people pictures of your kid, less is always more.

And so this is for the people who would love passionately to get their foot into the door of Planet Television and don't want me to skip straight to the sex and gossip. For everyone else, I would skim-read the next bit but there won't be any sex and gossip later because working in documentaries is essentially eating a sausage roll on the motorway at 1 a.m.

On the night I had my Road to Damascus Career Moment all I knew about the work world was that my job as a marketing assistant was sodding boring and life after university was pretty depressing. Very much living for the weekends, I skipped along to my friend Eugenie's house party and, having drunk lots of Smirnoff Ice, I was mooching about chatting to people I didn't know and occasionally winding my hips to Salt-N-Pepa until, as always happens at parties, everyone gradually gathered in the kitchen and started raiding the cupboards in search of salt and pepper Hula Hoops.

It was here that I found myself chatting to someone or other in a bit of a boozy daze when he told me that he was a television director.

Me:   A what?

Boy:  A television director. I make documentaries for television.

Me:   A *what?*! That's a real job that people our age do and that pays you real money and that's what you spend every day doing?

Call me a twonk but it had never occurred to me that this might be a possible career option. And, I am embarrassed to admit this, I even did a media module at university, where my friend Polly and I wrote, produced, directed and edited a trailer for a (fictional) detective series. But, being a complete plonker, even though I had loved every minute of the project, I hadn't joined the dots and I hadn't given a second's thought to how I could transfer that love and enjoyment into a job.

But as the director described what his job actually involved, I knew this was the one for me. Everything about it made me want to do a little dance. I loved the idea of handling the cameras and kit, I loved the idea of being on the road, travelling around to find great stories, meeting weird and wonderful people and then disappearing into an edit suite to eat biscuits and put the footage together like a brilliant puzzle.

And so I Googled the bejesus out of the industry and decided that I needed to hand in my resignation at my depressing marketing job and get work experience, preferably at the mothership, the BBC. When I told people of my plan there was a resounding 'It's so competitive, you'll never get in, they're firing people in the industry, they're making cutbacks . . .', and because I was young and thankfully naive, I thought, *Well, someone has to make telly, because it's on every day and every night and so why can't that someone be me?* So I went for it like a dog eating hot chips.

I took so much care over my work-experience application that it was the first thing the production manager mentioned. I think they thought I was a bit sad as I'd pretty much written a dissertation about why they should accept me into their love nest. And so I was given work experience at the Beeb (it can take two or three attempts at applying before being given a placement so if you really want it keep going) and I was as happy as a clam. I then promptly moved back home, bought some Tupperware for packed lunches and accepted that I would be entirely broke but entirely happy.

Just before I started I was given some excellent advice by my brother's girlfriend. She told me that no matter what job I was doing, I should do my absolute best. Whether it was sweeping up rubbish, or making a cup of tea, or opening mail, I should take pride in it and do it brilliantly. And this was a gem. Because work-experience bods come and go quickly and it takes a lot to make an impression in the short month that you're allowed in the building. As a tiny fish in a huge sea, all you have is your ability to make people's lives easier. I didn't know anything about production or filming or kit or editing. But I did know how to get crew lunch quickly or how to make sure there were extra crisps in the office on a busy day or how to reorganize the tape shelf without being asked or how to spend an entire evening, until the security guard kicked me out, tidying the props cupboard (it was huge and everyone always complained that they couldn't find anything within its hell-vortex). I remember once being asked to hold a door open as one of the live programmes wanted to film a presenter running down the corridor. And I held that door open for two hours. And even though a tin of paint could have done the same job, I felt that it was something of a test (it wasn't, they just wanted the door to be held open) and I wanted to show the universe how much I wanted a job.

This all sounds very brown-nosey and quite desperate, but work experience was only four weeks long so I threw my pride out of the window and threw everything at the job and tried to make myself indispensable. And I loved every minute of it because I was at the actual real BBC. And every day I walked through reception with nothing short of joy in my heart.

I was then made a correspondence assistant for the show I was working on. It was a *real* job paid in *real* money. I worked in television! And that was one of the most fun jobs I will probably ever have. I sat with four other correspondence assistants opening the letters that kids had written and we replied to them. We were in our own office with little to no manager presence and, whilst we worked very hard, we also played very hard. During our lunch breaks we would mooch about the famous BBC doughnut (which was in the old television centre in White City). We once bumped into David Dimbleby rehearsing for the election coverage and bought him an ice lolly. Another time we happened upon a hoard of *Star Wars* Stormtroopers and helped them find Studio One. At the end of one particularly long day opening mail, I left the office only to find Beyoncé performing a free concert in the car park.

And because I opened letters extremely well, I was promoted to correspondence assistant at *Blue Peter*. Which was beyond exciting. I was in charge of sending out the famous, precious *Blue Peter* badges. Again my job was to go through the letters and paintings and macaroni pictures sent in by thousands and thousands of children across the country and dish out the appropriate badges and response letters. The deal was if you worked like a monster and ploughed through enormous sacks of mail, you would be rewarded by joining the filming team on an excursion. Genius. So I would come in an hour before everyone and work like a beast until I was given the chance to go out on a real film shoot. And standing in the rain, manning the second camera, up to my knees in mud and with four more hours to go, I knew I was happy and had perhaps found the right job for me.

The next few years were a whirlwind of running about being the keenest bean of a runner this side of the Atlantic. I learned about cameras, I booked endless cabs, I became an expert at who liked what hot drink, I learned the basics of editing and how the commissioning process worked and how to find a giant plastic rat at 8 p.m. on a Friday. I learned that, as a runner with little to no television skills, my currency was making shit happen. I learned that, no matter how random or bonkers or unachievable the task, you always smiled and said, 'Yes, of course,' and only when they were out of earshot did you have a gigantic meltdown. And, because the internet had been born and I was in the middle of London, there was always, always a solution. So, gradually and slowly but surely, I went from runner to researcher to assistant producer, loving every minute.

OK not every minute but many, many minutes. I have a very rose-tinted memory of those times. There were of course moments when I was so tired I wanted to crawl under the desk and sleep for ever. I remember one particularly busy production, a little like *Faking It* for kids, when I worked fourteen-hour days for a two-week stretch, driving the crew backwards and forwards between London and Birmingham to save money on hotels, and then once I'd dropped everyone at their homes, going back to the office to put all the kit into the storeroom and recharge all the camera batteries, getting into bed at around 1 a.m. And then I would return to the office at 5 a.m. the next day to start it all again. I remember being so insane with tiredness that I burst into tears in my boyfriend's shower, but all I could think about whilst I was crying was that it was taking up valuable sleeping time, which would make me cry again, and I knew I was probably at the end of my proverbial tether. But I was so hungry to move up the food chain I just dug deep and found the energy to carry on. It was brilliant preparation for having a newborn baby.

However, mostly it was a wonderful time. Then one day, a producer friend of mine mentioned that BBC Three were looking for an immersive journalist and, having observed how nosey I was, suggested I try out for the job. That evening, almost just for something funny to do, he set up the office camera and we made a tape. And because he Gets Shit Done, it was edited and sent by the following morning. Amazing. And, after a few weeks, BBC Three replied and said they'd like a meeting. It was such a scary moment getting the lift to the sixth floor, where all the big bosses had their offices – somewhere, even though I had now worked at the BBC for four years, I had never been. The meeting was with Danny Cohen, who was running the channel at the time, and a commissioner, Harry Lansdown. Obviously I tried to be cool and nonchalant but inside I was fucking terrified. White cold terror. Which I know is not cool but it is the truth. And to cut a long story short, they must have decided I was bonkers enough to make a TV show. And they commissioned *Drinking with the Girls*, which I absolutely loved filming. For the next three months I travelled around the UK, unsurprisingly drinking with the girls, investigating women's relationship with alcohol from the youngest drinker to the eldest. And this was how I got into presenting. And the only difference between being in production and being on the telly was that I had to put on mascara before I came to work. Other than that, it was the same Ginsters pasty from a service station, the same silly car games when stuck in traffic, the same five layers of thermals. I loved it.

## My Yearly Plan

As a freelancer, I have to give myself an appraisal and I sometimes even take myself for away days. This year I am going to take myself for an office party with a cracker and a hat (oh God, that is so sad I could cry). Whilst I adore the freedom of being my own boss and working in a trendy café rather than doing a nine to five, I really miss the camaraderie of an office. I miss Friday-night drinks, I miss getting inappropriately drunk with Sue from Finance and talking rubbish with Bob from IT, and I miss singing 'Happy Birthday' slowly (and always slightly resembling a funeral march) to some poor sod who has to pretend that they are surprised by the party in the meeting room as everyone stands awkwardly in a semi-circle, eating Colin the Caterpillar cake from M&S and bowls of cheesy crisps, secretly gagging to get back to their desks so they can carry on instant-messaging Bob from IT. OK, I don't miss the birthday parties, but I do miss the other bits.

So, back to appraisals. Below is one of my absolute favourite work techniques, a beautiful gift from a wonderful ex-boss. In the olden days I used to write my Life Wish List thus:

- I want to understand my tax
- I want to take Coco ice skating
- I want to try Five Rhythms
- I want to visit my godmother
- I want to learn how to make homemade tacos
- I want to understand what's going on in *Game of Thrones*

I was saying to the universe that 'I wanted' to do these things. And, from past experience, that's what happens. I continue to *want* those things. I never actually *achieve* them. It's as though the universe is a huge mirror and it reflects back to us what we show it. We say 'want' and so that's what the universe delivers. So I have now changed my list and it looks like this:

- I understand my tax
- I take Coco ice skating

- I try Five Rhythms
- I visit my godmother
- I learn how to make homemade tacos
- I never understand *Game of Thrones* because that's not possible

In one month I have understood my finances, I have taken Coco ice skating, I haven't (yet) been to Five Rhythms, and I have visited my godmother in Essex. The tacos were awful but at least it's a start. I've got thirteen days left this month and I feel confident that I will complete the list. I mean, and this is directed to the universe, 'I complete the list.' Right. Now I have probably made at least twenty per cent of the five people reading this think I am a total nutcase. But even so, I promise, at the very least, it's worth trying. And then sharing with people you don't mind thinking you're a nutcase.


## A Very Public Bad Day At Work

Of course even the best jobs can go hideously wrong sometimes. We've all had those days – when the train is delayed and you get shouted at for being late, then the deal/project/presentation you've been working on goes tits up, then you drift off in a meeting and your evil boss asks you a question and you have that bottom-clenching realization that you have literally no idea what she's talking about, then Dave from the post room makes a 'hilarious' comment about your arse as you walk past . . . Well, you get the picture. I don't think there's a woman or man amongst us who hasn't had to nip to the loos and have a little weep at work from time to time.

Sadly, unlike riding a bike or making a homemade taco or child-rearing, there is no YouTube tutorial on how to deal with making a shit television series. This has happened to me and it is pretty horrendous. Firstly, even if the outcome is a bit poo, it still took the same blood, sweat and tears to make. And, in my experience, the ones that don't work are the hardest to make because, somewhere along the line, everyone starts to get that sinking feeling that it's just not working. And so the hours become longer, the pressure intensifies and the atmosphere becomes extremely challenging because everyone really wants to stop making it and go home. But you've signed the contract, you've booked the days and there is no way off the train.

So you just have to dig in and do your absolute best. And then, when it's over, it is part of my job to talk about how very wonderful it is on the radio and in newspapers and on breakfast television. When the programme is good this is one of the most fun parts of my job. And if the programme is not good, then it is truly painful. It's hard to describe but the closest I can get is that it leaves me feeling extremely naked. That's what I get paid for – in part – to take the shit. But, regardless, it's not very nice and I don't have very thick skin. I have papier-mâché skin – it looks solid but it's not. But whether it's a crap TV show or a marketing presentation that you weren't prepared for or a finance report that doesn't add up, everyone has experienced work humiliation. The question is how to deal with it? Because the real test of being a human is how you cope when all you want to do is crawl back into bed. And, for me, the only technique that works is going back to my centre. I used to hear that phrase bandied about and I didn't really understand it but I interpret it as the feeling you get when you turn off your phone, take a moment to be quiet (totally easy with two kids) and try to get a sense of peace. If I'm ever able to do this, it gives me a sense of perspective and the issue suddenly doesn't feel like such an issue. I achieve this at least 2 out of 100 times. And if that isn't possible then I self medicate with real three-dimensional humans and gin. They are the ones who can remind us that work, and the success/failure of our professional life, is not who we are and not indicative of our value as a human being. So I call my mum or my friends and have a moan and maybe a little cry and a laugh, maybe pop into Topshop and buy some new shorts and then, gradually, start to feel better. And tomorrow the sting will be a little less. And then, in my case, a new, more awful programme will come out, and suddenly no one cares about your small stain on television history. Because they are too busy writing/talking/tweeting about something else. This is the beauty and pain of life – it just carries on. The world keeps turning and the past falls away from us and all we can do is resist the temptation to hide, be brave, stand straight, fix anything we can, say sorry if we need to, call the people that love us and try to learn from what happened. If you can master that then you deserve a certificate.

## *Brain Food*

I use my brain nearly every day for vital tasks such as how to work my remote control and how to open children's toys (why are they wrapped in plastic and ties so thick it takes a circular saw to free them?) and how to make kale not taste like punishment. So, in order for it to assist me in these great life predicaments, I am trying to nourish it. I wasn't so aware of the importance of this when I was younger but the older I get the more conscious I am of what I'm feeding my brain.

By this I mean what messages we choose to absorb, which values we pick up and transmit to others in turn. Because there is a mean worm inside all of us. I'm not saying we've all got worms – although I have had worms a few times – but rather that there is something inside us that shouldn't be encouraged. A bit like road rage, it's there inside us and we can either choose to feed it or take a deep breath and not rise to it. I'm not sure how I went from brain to worms to driving but let me rein in the metaphors and return to reality.

Which takes me nicely on to reality magazines. When I say reality magazines, I mean utterly-fictional-not-what-life-should-be-about magazines. This is where an entire publication is given over to whether a reality star has lost three pounds and looks good in her yellow bikini on holiday. Or whether another reality star has been 'unlucky in love', and we are invited to join in faux-sympathy whilst clearly the magazine itself is revelling in (and directly profiting from) this woman's misery. Or imposing pity on them, the biggest offenders being weight and romantic status, when they are probably completely content with being brilliant at their chosen field and don't want to starve themselves or put a ring on it.

It's like we're made up of so many different appetites, and we can choose to feed or starve different parts of ourselves – and these magazines feed a not-very-nice side of our beings. It's the side that compares ourselves to other women, that thinks we are what we can afford to buy, that judges someone on where they go on holiday or how cool their shoes are. In our right mind we know that these are puerile views but if we're often absorbing them, it's hard to remember that. I sometimes hate how much of a hypocrite I can be. I know that it's horrible to judge people for how they look, yet when I walk down the street my internal narrative can be so judgemental – looking at how well they are dressed, or not, how cool they look – and I catch myself doing it and wonder what the fuck is going on. How can my stated beliefs and principles be so counter to what's actually happening in my head?

And that's when I give myself a media audit. What shows have I been watching? Who have I been hanging out with? What have I been reading? Although individually they aren't bad – reading one celeb magazine in a hairdresser isn't going to destroy your peace of mind for ever – the cumulative effect of pinging from celeb magazines to pop programmes to mean chat in the pub creates the person that we are inside. We can talk about women's true value and the deeper, truer confidence that a woman can have until we're blue in the face but until we are living it and thinking it it's all a bunch of arse.

So it's about being *for* each other. It's about celebrating women's successes, their character, their achievements. This doesn't mean being Super Dooper Nice all the time – it's obviously fine to disagree, debate, dislike. But let's make sure it's not because we don't like their hair or think they're not the right shape or think they have crap shoes. If there is one subliminal way that misogyny will thrive, it's by constantly convincing us that women are mostly about what they look like. But they are not. We are not. God, I am not. My daughter is so much more. I love my friends and I hope they know the brilliance of themselves – not because their hair looks thick or because they have tight buttocks, but because they're kind and funny and interesting and thoughtful and just, well, themselves.

We as individuals have such a powerful ripple effect. If my friend questions something in the media, it makes me think; I tell another friend; it makes her think and so on and so on. And if the result of that questioning creates a better sense of self-worth, then the significance of passing it on and on and on is immense. Every time I check the *Daily Mail* online site, every time I read a crap celeb magazine and criticize someone's bikini body, it's like I am giving in to my worm – and, whether we like it or not, our thoughts and actions *do* affect others because we are not islands (unless you are a mute that lives on an island).

I've always thought it was quite lame to always blame the media for the world's problems. And, on the whole, it *is* lame. But when it comes to women's sense of self-worth there is something hard to deny: after I've read the *Mail Online*, I feel a very subtle but very real sense of self-hatred ('If that's how disgusting they find her cellulite, they would find me a hideous monster') and, if I'm not being conscious, I carry that competitive, shallow, mean perception into my view of other women. Hate breeds hate. And I don't want that going on inside of me.

Luckily the more I realize the adverse effect it has on me, the easier it becomes to resist the temptation. Like cigarettes. I used to think they were lush, and then I found out – really, really found out, thanks to a programme I made that took me to a hospital lung cancer ward – how they disintegrate your precious lungs and every single one destroys the fragile fibres inside you. Now it's easier not to have one (just for the record, I do sometimes, because I am a numpty). In the same way, the more I see how those anti-women sites and mags affect me, the easier it is to leave them on the shelf. And that's when that overused phrase 'spreading awareness' really means something. Because sometimes just being aware is ninety-nine per cent of the solution.

# 4. Letter to My Heart: Love, Heartbreak, the Lady Family, Relationships

*Dearest Heart,*

*Wow, where do I start? I am honestly stumped. I feel like the shy girl in the movies who has so much to say to the boy she loves that she ends up saying nothing at all and staring at her trainers. I feel like I should be composing a beautiful poem but I am terrible at writing poetry (having learned the hard way by trying to write raps during my twenties and performing them as spoken word – yeah, that happened; please can we now never mention it ever again, ever? Thank you).*

*You are the only body part that I sometimes wish functioned less efficiently. Which sounds insane as I eat my greens and do my cardio and generally try to make sure you are feeling grrreat. But sometimes I wish you had a dimmer switch. I don't want to be a robot but the ferocity with which you exercise your rainbow of emotions is sometimes hard to keep up with.*

*When I am heartbroken it can feel like you are hungry or imploding or have run out of fuel or are trying to escape from my chest or trying to change shape or becoming both a balloon and a shrivelled raisin or maybe even crawling very slowly from my chest up into my windpipe and out of my mouth, like the reverse of swallowing a huge, bitter, aching pill. They say it's better to have loved and lost than never to have loved at all, but buggery bollocks, it's hard to agree with this when you're in the thick of it.*

*Being in love feels like you are expanding or exploding or covered in Deep Heat or plugged into the mains or standing on the top of a cliff on a sunny day with the breeze in your hair or like you have a tiny supernova about to break forth from your ribs. It makes you want to listen to Phil Collins and dance all day and kiss the faces of strangers and learn how to speak Spanish and make muffins and run to Bristol.*

*Of course I don't really want you to be subdued. Because with the intense romantic heartbreak that feels like my innards have been hit by a gigantic invisible hammer comes the other extreme of butterfly-rave love and the huge, beautiful, uncomplicated, unconditional love for my kids. Yeah, they can drive me to shout profane language into my scarf whilst buying milk, but they also make me feel a love that is so simple and powerful that at some points I worry I might bite one of them.*

*So bosh on. Grow and implode and go cold and then burn, because when it gets too intense I have white wine and friends. Thank. God.*

## Love

### First Infatuation

My first real human crush, as opposed to that which causes furious licking of posters on a bedroom wall (Johnny Depp, Brad Pitt, Bros, Michael J. Fox), was on my first bestest friend, Lucy. I met her when I was six and instantly knew that this human was formidable. Even though she was so little, she had incredible charisma and charmed every teacher and student without even breaking a sweat. She was fun, complicated, moody, spontaneous, naughty, kind, selfish and always interesting. She lived in a thatched cottage on a disused farm with her wonderful mum, Sally, a goat that terrified me and an insane spaniel called Piper, who always looked like he was running from the police. She also had two older brothers who were only marginally less scary than the goat but who were a reliable source of beer and cigarettes (though not when we were six).

I even broke my female-sexual-experience cherry with Lucy. Having watched hours and hours of *Home and Away*, we thought it would be fun to try kissing, as all they ever seemed to do in Summer Bay was to try to land a kiss or kiss or talk about being kissed. So one night, when Lucy was sleeping over at my house, we got a flannel and put it between our mouths and gave it a whirl. I didn't have a sense of it being naughty but, at the same time, we never, ever talked about it either with each other or anyone else, so there must have been some idea that it wasn't the 'done thing'. It was only much later when I bumped into her in east London, having not seen each other for fifteen years, that we went for a drink and a walk down memory lane. And, having reflected on my sexual experiences for a TV documentary I had just made, I brought our 'kiss' up, as I wasn't sure whether it was something I had imagined. But she also remembered it and we laughed our arses off as we pieced our collective memories together and realized that neither of us had talked about it, or really thought about it, for over a decade. But yes, the flannel snogging had definitely happened.

## First Boy Crush

My first boy crush was called Tom. I was nine, and he was ten and a friend of my brother's. I remember going with my parents to watch my brother play cricket and being pant-wettingly excited that I got to see My One True Love (who I had never actually spoken to). And I made a total tit of myself. I didn't realize it at the time but this kind of thing was to become a regular experience in my romantic life. At half-time all the boys came to sit on the blanket to chomp on the Quavers and ham sandwiches that my mum had brought and, lo and behold, Tom planted his bottom next to mine. I nearly passed out. And to channel this tidal wave of love, I decided to joke around with the strange piece of cricket equipment that had been thrown on to the blanket. I joked that it was hard to imagine what this 'funny piece of plastic' was for. 'Is it a hat?' I said as I popped it on my head; 'Is it an elbow pad?' as I put it on my elbow; 'Or a gas mask?' as I put it over my mouth. At which point my brother did a commando roll and snatched it from me. But it was too late. Yes, I quickly learned that this little piece of plastic is called a 'box' and is used to protect boys' willies from the cricket ball. Tom didn't find me putting my brother's used box over my face an immediate catalyst for asking me out. Quite the opposite it seems. They thought it was hilarious. I did not. I am still not really over that.

## First Snog

It was New Year's Eve and my aunt and uncle were having a party at their home. I was wearing bright red gingham leggings, my Garfield T-shirt and my very best crushed velvet jacket. I was ready to party. And when I say party, what I mean is being herded upstairs so that the grown-ups could get on with eating and drinking and guffawing. There were about ten kids, ranging from ten years old (me) to fifteen (my cousin and his friends). We mucked about playing classic New Year's Eve games, such as charades and seeing how much of the grown-up punch the older boys could steal from downstairs.

About halfway through the evening I found myself in my cousin's bedroom alone with a boy called James. He was fifteen, good-looking, extremely cocky and very drunk. One minute we were talking about my cousin's NASA spaceship poster and the next he pounced. Suddenly he was snogging my face with the ferocity of a hungry lion ravaging a newly killed deer, which was mildly exciting but mostly massively scary.

I had never kissed a boy. I had never held a boy's hand. At this point my great romance had been with Michael J. Fox, in my head. But here I was, doing that snogging thing that I'd seen so many times on *Home and Away*. It was strange and he smelt strange and it made me feel strange. I didn't know what to do with my tongue or my body. So I decided to make like a sack of potatoes and just keep still.

And then it was over.

I walked, a bit dazed, into the playroom where everyone else was watching *Mary Poppins*. I was startled as I didn't really know what had just happened or whether I was in trouble or whether it was OK to feel weird about it or what who how when why. So I sat down and watched Dick Van Dyke jig about with penguins.

Then James came in. And he sat on the floor next to me and put his hand on my thigh for the rest of the film *like we'd been a couple for years*. Again, it was all so new and intimidating that I struggled to know how to react. So I didn't react. I just sat there like a statue.

And then James, having drunk a lot of punch, left the room and was sick out of the bathroom window and on to the conservatory where all the adults were having an elegant dinner.

And that was my first kiss.

James subsequently sent me four love letters, which was very weird but quite exciting, and even though the whole kiss thing had been really scary I cherished them as though we were Romeo and Juliet.

# First Puppy Love

My first experience of love – well, puppy love – was with the most beautiful boy I had ever seen at that point, Duncan. Oh wow. I remember climbing the stairs to my friend Char's bedroom, turning the corner and hearing a chorus of angels break into Handel's *Messiah* as I spotted a being of such brown-skinned, big-eyed beauty that it will forever be etched into my brain.

He was smokin'. And for some reason, even though I was wearing my mum's old silky Chinese kimono, platform patent-red trainers and multiple little buns in my hair (aka nineties Björk), he thought I was all right. I had double train-tracks – the sexy kind that are connected with colourful rubber bands and hooks – and spots. Plus I was loud and couldn't hold my alcopops. But I think this was exactly why he liked me. He was reserved and shy and I was the yin to his yang. I am just assuming this, as it certainly wasn't for my sense of style.

As for me, I felt as passionately for him as my underdeveloped sixteen-year-old heart had the capacity to feel. He was more mature than me in this area and I think he felt actual real love. But because I didn't understand this feeling I was not careful with his heart. Which I regret. And, having subsequently had my heart pulverized, I now know I behaved carelessly. I think, during our three-year relationship, I broke up with him five times, one of those being via a text message. I have since apologized to him.

But mostly we had a lovely relationship. He was peaceful and kind and fun and interesting and reliable. He didn't play games like so many other boys did and always called and turned up when he said he would. And so I will always be thankful to him for setting a positive precedent for future relationships.

## First Love

It was only when I fell in love that I realized the difference between massively liking someone and loving someone. It's as indefinable and yet as clear as the difference between feeling tired and feeling hungry. There are moments when they almost feel the same but, really, they are very different.

I met Janusz on a beach in Thailand when I was nineteen when the friend I was travelling with kissed the person he was travelling with, and it just seemed so convenient to hook up with him because then we could all hang out. Yeah, it was a fling entirely initiated by ease of logistics. And so we spent the evening together on a beach, drinking buckets of Thai whisky and Thai Red Bull (which is not like European Red Bull – there is something very different in it, plus it looks like cough medicine) and we almost certainly discussed the meaning of life and what bark is made of.

He seemed nice. He was Polish–Canadian with tattoos and a love of motorbikes, and he was completely different from any of the boys I'd grown up with. Intrigue turned to enjoyment, which then turned to a crush, which then turned to a huge crush, which quickly turned into raging, heart-pounding, nostril-flaring love. Because it caught me off-guard (how can it happen any other way?) and because it was my first time, it was almost oppressively powerful. I now know that is sometimes a bittersweet consequence of falling in love.

Thankfully for my friend, her trip was coming to an end and she was able to remove herself from her fling, who she had started to find very annoying, and also remove herself from Janusz and me, who had also started to be very annoying. But I still had a few weeks left of my travelling time so I continued to follow him around like a love-sick puppy. It was possibly one of the most magical few weeks of my life. At the time, any thought about the risk of travelling around with someone I barely knew was completely ignored. And any thought about the risk of driving around small island roads on a huge motorbike, wearing only a pair of shorts, a T-shirt and some flip-flops, was also completely ignored. And any thought about the risk of moving around without telling anyone at home where I was, was also completely ignored. Now, as a parent, I salute my mum and dad for giving me such glorious freedom and trust. I hope that I can do the same for my daughter, although I now appreciate how incredibly hard that must have been.

Over ten years on and it's almost impossible to say why Janusz was my first love. Yes, I found him incredibly attractive, and he was open, interesting, energetic, unusual, kind and much more. But there are many people like that. Even now I don't know what makes people fall in love – it's indefinable – which is why love is so scary and exciting. It is intoxicating, powerful and primal. When my money ran out I flew home, got a job stacking shelves in Sainsbury's and saved up enough to buy a ticket to Australia (where he had gone) to stay with him. I would have done anything and gone anywhere to see him again. Every yoghurt I placed on to those freezing shelves was placed with enthusiasm and love, knowing it was taking me one step closer to seeing his face. Sickening, I know. Unbearably cheesy. Vomitingly naff. But this is what loves does. It turns you into a crazy person.

And whilst I know that the heart is just a red squidgy organ that pumps blood around our body, I also can't deny that the feeling of love comes firmly from where it sits. It definitely doesn't come from our brain. Or even our fanny. When my heart is broken, the pain is where my heart is and when I am emanating love it comes from the same place. And when the person I love is on their way, it's my heart that beats so hard and so fast that it might pop out of my ribcage and flop on to the table like a suffocating fish. When we are madly in love, our whole body is infected – almost weakened – but it most definitely starts from our heart.

It was only when I experienced this feeling that I really understood why so many songs, almost all of them, are about love. I used to think (and still do) it was bonkers that there is such a lack of variety in song topics. Why not write a song about how annoying automated checkouts are (no, I haven't put a fucking unidentified object in the basket) or how it feels to be promoted or how great it feels to repaint a room or how depressing it can be to open a letter from HMRC? All of these things are common experiences and rouse strong emotion – so why not write about them? It's like there is a secret songwriting code and they make a promise that they'll only write about finding love, losing love, sex, smoking pot and making money. Anything else is, apparently, bollocks.

But then I fell in love and realized that the reason ninety-five per cent of songs and poetry and stories and opera and spoken word (shudder) and theatre is about love is because when it happens, or when it leaves you, your world stops and everything else fades into insignificance. The power, the passion, is so intense that it might even inspire you to put pen to paper and write some poetry or even, God help us, spoken word. Because no matter how scared I am when I get a letter from HMRC, or how much I love baked beans, nothing even comes close to the blood-draining, eye-rolling, skin-melting feeling of being in love with someone. It's euphoric and shattering and wonderful and devastating.

That's how I felt about Janusz. But no matter how knee-tremblingly I felt about him, the world carried on turning. And my time was up and university was starting. I had worked extremely hard to get a place there and I knew that I had to go back to London. By this time Janusz and I, having lived and worked in Sydney for three months in a house with five other Aussie boys (larks), had spent two blissful weeks travelling up the coast. We had ended up in a hideous bug-infested hotel in Cairns as we had run out of money. And as the weirdest, most inappropriate parting gift of all time, I decided to spend my last few dollars on a huge cooked breakfast for him. I walked miles in some awful wooden clogs that gave me massive blisters to the supermarket in the blinding heat and, perhaps mad with heatstroke, chose to cook him steak and eggs for breakfast. Yeah.

So I hobbled back to our hostel and, whilst he was still asleep, went to the pool house where there was a stove, black with grease, and cooked for him. Beyoncé once sang about being 'crazy in love' but I'm not even sure she would understand this. And, of course, when Janusz woke up and saw this feast, his face said it all. Because he was kind, he sat down and made enthusiastic noises. But, like being slapped awake from sleepwalking, I immediately returned to the world of the sane and realized that I had done a very weird thing.

Anyway, he poked at the food and I was embarrassed and we got through it. And then he took me to the bus station to say goodbye so I could travel for twelve hours back to Sydney. Which, after spending the last of my money on steak and eggs and not having a bean to even buy a bean and feeling like my insides were going to fall out of my body because the pain was so bad, wasn't great. I remember the parting vividly – we hugged, we kissed, he said he would come to the UK (I knew he would never come to the UK), he said he was going to marry me (I knew we wouldn't get married), and he said he would spend the rest of his life with me (I suspected we would never see each other again). And then he walked away and I literally crawled into a corner and cried, wailing like an animal with an arrow in its bottom.

Then I scraped myself up and got on to the bus. And, after an hour or three of staring out of the window and crying into my scarf, I started talking to the girl sitting next to me. And she gave me some perspective by telling me she had travelled to Cairns to have an abortion because she was so scared her mean father would find out she had become pregnant and would beat her. So I stopped feeling sorry for myself.

Janusz and I never did see each other again. For a few months we emailed and chatted on the phone, but, by this time, I was getting up early to go to lectures and had a busy schedule and a new job and new friends and so being phoned at 3 a.m. by a stoned Canadian quickly became quite annoying. And having pined for him, I started to screen his calls. Wow, how quickly young love cometh and goeth . . .

# Heartbreak

## First Heartbreak

So when I say 'first heartbreak', what I should really say is 'first stomach-churning rejection'. Saying goodbye to Janusz at the bus station had given me my first delightful experience of feeling like my heart had actually dissolved. Whilst it was intensely painful at the time, I'm glad I didn't know that it gets worse, otherwise I might have decided to become a nun. They say that sticks and stones may break your bones but words will never hurt you – but they are talking crap. Sticks and stones hurt but you can put some Savlon on your wounds and someone might even give you a lolly. Emotional hurt is much harder to get over and, in some cases, leaves deeper scars than any physical wound.

Even now, a decade later, I can still feel the sensation of someone sucking the air and blood and organs from my chest as Kevin delivered the news that he didn't want me. We had been on–off together for a few years at university and swung from being friends to being in a relationship to being friends until I realized that I was bone-deep in love with him. So I told him. And he said that he would have to think about it. Righto. And, because we were at a small drama school, we saw each other every day, often in intense environments, which is fantastic when you're desperately in love with someone who is weighing up whether they want to be with you. There is no room for a bad-hair day in that situation. Because my timing is excellent I had dropped this bomb on him just after we had committed to being in a two-person play, set in a tent, with two months of rehearsal before the performance. (I was studying drama and education, not acting, so to make matters worse this was entirely voluntary and did not contribute to my final mark.) So, for at least an hour a day, I was cheek-to-cheek with him, sometimes secretly smelling his neck and hoping he wouldn't notice and think I was creepy, all the while wondering, waiting for his answer. At several points during our lovely little intense play in the tent he would crawl out to deliver a monologue and I would have to try not to bite his bum.

So I waited and I tried not to scream 'Just tell me' in his face every day and be mature and give him space. Sometimes being mature is like pulling teeth. For a while, life carried on as normal. We spent most of our time together, and when he was bored he would come round to my flat and we would laugh together and go to parties together and dance. When I say dance, I mean Kevin would unroll his piece of lino and we would breakdance with the other 'breakers' (I can't get away with saying that now without sounding like a proper twonk so I'm afraid it has to go in inverted commas) in our 'crew' (help me). My breakdance name was Wily Kit, you know, like from *Thundercats*, and at one point I had a bandana with sewn-on braids that I actually wore and not as a joke. I was the love child of Axl Rose and Jay Z. OK, moving on, and that's never to be mentioned ever again until I'm drunk at a wedding and show you my moves.

But I mention the dancing because it was partly why I could not fathom not having Kevin as my One True Love. Because he was one in a million and I knew that people like that don't come around very often. Whenever I describe him, it's as 'the Northern Irish breakdancing born-again Christian'. Boom. And he more than lived up to the excitement and interest and surprise of his introduction. One of his most attractive qualities was how he made everyone feel special – he would always notice the people on the periphery of a party or gathering and make sure they were OK. If they weren't having a good time, he would make sure they were included in the fun. And because he was so extraordinarily confident and charismatic and clever, he was often the heart of the party but never tried to be cool or elusive because he was naturally cool and being elusive is so deeply boring.

I know this must sound like I am just blowing smoke up his bum but I wanted to lay it out because I knew that this person was a bit of a diamond. Which is why I felt like I had been shot when, three months later, Kevin called me. It was during the Christmas holidays and I was sitting on the sofa, feeling grey, watching *Friends* (slippery slope). The phone in the kitchen rang and it was him. And he told me that, having thought about it for a long time, he didn't want to be with me. Even though I was half expecting it, it hit me like someone punching me in the stomach. It was incredibly physical and I had to hold on to the side of the kitchen worktop to stop myself falling over as my legs buckled. I can remember not really being able to speak and also feeling bad for making him do all the talking because what could he possibly say to make it better?

The next six months was a blur of cereal and back-to-back *Friends*. I would not recommend this to anyone as a good way to self-medicate but at least it's marginally better than tequila or crack. I know that most people have felt acute heartbreak, but I was blindsided at how low and grey and flat and bleak it was. It was like a great big depressed slug had made a home where my heart had once been and every day it became bigger and more attached and I wondered if I'd ever lark or frolic about again.

Because I had recovered from the pain of parting with Janusz in less time than it takes to make a Pot Noodle, I was slightly expecting to be done by the time Monday rolled around. But it dragged on and on until I had forgotten how to interact with three-dimensional people or what it was like to eat food that didn't come out of a cardboard box.

So this is how I spent my Christmas holiday and, when university started again, I told Kevin that I couldn't see him at all. Because every time I was within fifty feet of him, the giant slug wailed like it had slurped on a salt milkshake. Every time he did a head-spin my insides would do a dry-spin (sorry, had to do a breakdancing pun at some point). Like an addict, I knew that the only way to reha-bilitate was to go cold turkey. It was the only way to surgi-cally remove the Slug of Pain.

This was also greatly helped by my friend Polly, who swooped in and staged a much-needed intervention. She removed my left hand from the cereal box, she removed my right hand from the telly remote and removed my chin from the floor. Polly reminded me that it might be nice to have a bath and wash my hair, and perhaps even leave the house occasionally. Gradually I moved from elasticated waistbands to jeans and from watching other people live their life on telly to actually living mine in reality.

It took me about two years to fully get over him. Which I slightly carry like a badge of honour, as though it qualifies me as a true member of the human race. YES, I have had my heart blown to smithereens; YES, I have loved and lost; YES, I understand what Phil Collins is singing about.

## Worst Date

Unfortunately my worst-ever date came immediately after my worst-ever heartbreak. At that time I was working the evening shift at Somerset House where, every winter, they put up an ice rink. The cloakroom was in a little portable shed with a heater, with a good supply of KitKats and five broke students taking care of people's precious belongings. It was a hoot, and exactly what I needed as it removed the risk of bumping into Kevin at the student union and helped me crawl my way out of my three-grand credit-card debt.

This is where I met Ben. He was silly, warm and made the shift go quickly. He was also a hottie, which didn't hurt. They say that it's not a good idea to move immediately from one person to another, but I disagree. (OK, it's probably not a good idea to move from one serious relationship straight into another, although, even then, are we kidding ourselves that we can control the timing of meeting someone we like?) A stepping-stone romance is hugely helpful in unhooking our hearts from another person. And so there was Ben: tall, dark, handsome and as silly as a bumful of Smarties. Perfect.

So we laughed and checked coats and drank hot chocolate and it really took the edge off feeling broken inside. Not surprisingly I developed a huge crush on him. And then Ben asked me on a date and I was so happy I thought I might pop.

We arranged to meet at Covent Garden Tube station and go from there as he had some fun plans up his sleeve. And I thought, *Well, that bodes very well*, as I love it when a guy is assertive and thinks of things to do. So, wearing my new New Look purple jersey dress and adorned in my finest Topshop gold chain, I waited at the Tube station, trying to calm the butterflies having a rave in my abdomen. Then he appeared through the crowds of Italian tourists, a vision of stained dishevelment. He had chosen to wear his very best torn, dirty tracksuit bottoms and a T-shirt that smelt like a wet dog. His hair was greasy and I knew instantly that he was stoned. Flipping lovely.

Anyway, because I am British and polite, I smiled and didn't scream into his face that a shower wouldn't have gone amiss. Then we went on our adventure. His fun plan was mainly mooch-based and, as we proceeded on our Great Mooch, he told me about the various times he and his brother had been stoned, and the funny things they had talked about (much, much worse than seeing people's holiday photos) and how they had laughed this one time at this thing that happened but you had to be there. We mooched past the Institute of Contemporary Arts and mooched inside to find they were about to show a film about table tennis (it was actually quite good). He thought it would be really funny, especially as he was stoned.

We then wandered aimlessly out of the cinema and continued with our mooching. I gradually realized that the date was not going to get better. But rather than being assertive and going home, I continued to trail along alongside him because, at that time, I had not yet developed the power to say what I was actually feeling. So it went on.

Next on our agenda was food because Ben had the munchies, natch. So we drifted around until he found a newsagent's that sold samosas and he bought one whilst I waited outside. When he appeared he had already taken a gigantic bite out of the spicy parcel of grease and meat, and this is when he decided it was time for our first kiss. He lunged at me, giving me the full tonguey works, and I felt his hand on the back of my head. As he was still clutching the samosa, I was left with a lovely oily patch in my hair. And because he had not yet swallowed his mouthful, I was also given bits of lamb and pea and onion. Yes, this happened.

Even though I am British and polite there is a line and this was the line. So I made the excuse that I had to feed my cat and I left. Even though I had spent months swooning over him and thought he was as beautiful as the day is light, I never went on another date with him because I realized that I had just been on The Worst Date of All Time and one was probably enough.

But even though it had been The Worst Date of All Time, it served a valuable purpose and I had broken the dating ice after having not dated for many years. The only way was up.

### The Lady Family

I have loved dating, even with samosas and mooching, and I have loved the ups and down and ins and outs of romantic life. But I'm pretty sure that one of the main reasons I've enjoyed riding the love roller coaster so much is because of the stability I get from the Lady Family. Most girls have a lady family and I salute them all as I believe that this is one of the most important ways to ensure sanity and happiness and joy in your life.

Pretty much any positive adjective I could muster, they embody. In an unpredictable world, they are a constant. We have driven each other mad at various times in our twenty-year friendships, and had fallings-out and shouted at each other but, because it's not a romantic relationship, these never flare up so fiercely that it breaks the bond and we've always found a way back.

But now logistics are not on our side. We all have busy jobs and some of us have time-sucking babies and some of us have box-set addictions. In our twenties we went through a period of bailing on our plans to see each other. Then one of the group, who is extremely straight-talking, thankfully and rightly announced that she would no longer accept cancellations unless we were either dying or dead. Whilst that sounds stern, she was right. I was personally sick of turning up at their houses to find that they had left work an hour late or not at all. And I was sick of setting out to one of their houses to receive a text to say that they were 'really, really tired'. But I was doing it too. Having had them so conveniently close for such a long time, I hadn't quite clocked on to the fact that I had to make an effort. I might not be 'in the mood' but what if one of them really needed me that night? What was the message I was giving them? When it was winter and it got dark early and it was cold, it seemed like too much hard work to trudge across London to see them. After all, they'd be there tomorrow. But I learned (and am still learning) that friendships are like gardens – they need investment, they need time, they need love in order to grow and thrive. If you snooze, you lose.

Now we're in our mid-thirties our relationships have changed again. Even though there are more babies and longer working days and fancier job titles and bigger responsibilities, we see each other regularly and the bond feels even stronger. I wonder if that is because, unlike at school when we were all within arm's reach, we have consciously chosen each other. Life and work and circumstance could have easily moved us apart, but something has held us together like No More Nails. I think it's because we now see, in sharp relief, how important we are to each other. I don't want to get all cheesy but it's hard not to. I think we've understood how precious friendships are and how every minute of seeing each other, every phone call, every text – just touching base and showing our support and reassuring each other of our presence – means everything. Because, I think, when you reach your thirties, you realize that life doesn't turn out how you imagine. People you thought were perfect matches divorce. Careers you thought were ideal don't work out. The Disney fairy tale of riding off into the sunset with The One doesn't happen, nor does the picket fence, nor does the magical Fairy Godmother. And whilst real life is much more interesting and beautiful and exciting, it can also be much scarier, much tougher and much less predictable.

I remember one particular friend going through a divorce a few years ago. I was busy with a new job and I was excited about finally getting some experience holding a camera and shooting every single day. I kept missing her calls and, as I am terrible on the phone, never quite made the time to call her back. Because I was busy and she was busy I made some crappy excuse that life was making it tricky to be there for her. Bullshit. It was a simple matter of priorities. When you want to call someone, you make the time. When you want to see someone, you make the time. And ninety-nine per cent of the time, any excuse given for not being available at *some* point in the day is about priorities.

Unless you are a surgeon or an astronaut there really isn't an excuse for not replying to a text, other than it wasn't important to you. And I put my hands up to that. But I think I caught it just in time. I gave myself a talking-to, acknowledging that I had not been there for her and that I adored her and she was absolutely a priority to me and that I should show that through action not intention and that time waits for no woman. She was getting divorced *now*. Not in a month when my work contract was finished, but *now*. And I was either going to support her through it or I wasn't. No amount of intention was going to change that. That realization had a huge impact on me. I started calling her. Lots. And I am pathetically grateful for that revelation because I have needed her love and support myself many, many times since then.

Then there are the Big Decisions. And as life goes on, those decisions seem to get heavier and the fish you're frying get bigger and the stakes become higher and the ripples affect more people and are sometimes dramatically life-changing and terrifying. Without the Lady Family I don't know what I would do. Of course they can't make my choices for me but there is something invaluable about people you believe to be kind and wise and who know you inside and out, helping to guide you without any judgement. It's magic. I'd say that was pretty good value. Anyway. I love them. That is all.

## Relationships

As this book goes to print, the ink is only just drying on my divorce. It has been a bit like living in a snow globe – I still feel shaken up, but every day things get a little bit calmer and I'm now starting to see through the storm. Thankfully my ex and I have been able to go through this process in a calm and peaceful way, but of course it is really hard at times. As everything is still so raw, for now I'm going to keep things general on the topic of relationships.

I believe we should view relationships as something we work at and get better at. I feel sad when I hear so many married people tell me that they no longer feel cherished or appreciated by their partner. Commitment can provide such an amazingly strong sense of security, but it can also breed a sense of complacency. A little like sex, I used to think relationships happened entirely organically and naturally, and if it wasn't working then it just wasn't there. I now know that, if you actively choose, you can learn about how to be better at relationships and, if you're open and willing, then you can change and grow and have deeper, more intense, more intimate, more committed relationships than you ever thought possible.

Relationships, whether they last a month or five years or thirty-five, teach us so much about ourselves. It's like the other human holds a mirror up and you see things that you love and things that you don't love. Growing up, I realized that I could either learn from the bad things and change (which is *fantastically* hard), or carry on being a plonker. You also learn how to pick your battles, how to be calm when you feel like shouting, how to shout when you know you need to be heard and how love is a verb.

I was so excited the first time I lived with a boyfriend like an actual real grown-up and it was magical. It was a hoot and we would spend the evening on the sofa talking and the weekends shopping in markets for food to cook for our friends and I felt like I was in a film and it was utter bliss. But, every so often, my passive-aggressive monster would appear. Having never lived so intensely with just one person, I hadn't met my passive-aggressive self – but it was there and it was ugly.

I would storm off after something tiny happened, and refuse to answer phone calls or messages and fester in a nearby bar until we were both miserable. I didn't realize that was my intended outcome. As someone who struggles with upfront confrontation, I would use silence to express my upset. This is a terrible way to get what you want as, basically, you don't get what you want and both parties suffer. It's also the coward's way out because if someone questions you, because nothing has been said, it's possible to pretend that you're 'Fine – no, *really*!', thus prolonging the misery for all and never growing as a couple. Not good.

Thankfully I was never punished for doing this and I would return, often as pitifully as possible, soaking from walking in the rain, to open arms. But, even though my actions were knee-jerk and unconsciously performed, on one level I was aware of how bonkers and unfair they were. It was something I needed to get a grip of. So, with the help of my very patient boyfriend, I tried to stop it. Which was abstract and incredibly hard and like trying to remove a splinter using a spoon. But I learned my triggers (white wine) and also to identify the feeling that would propel me into the spiral of pain and passive-aggressive punishment. I learned that if I could catch it at *that* moment and openly voice how I was feeling in a very literal way, such as, 'I think I am about to go into my passive-aggressive black hole,' then it would break the spell and I would be able to dodge it. I also created the 'White Wine Rule' which prevented me from starting an intense, passive-aggressive conversation about our relationship, after white wine (well, any alcohol). This has gloriously prevented many, many unnecessary, stressful discussions/ arguments that I regret when I wake up. So, gradually, the more I shone a light on to the ridiculous behaviour, the quicker I was able to stop doing it. I felt very happy that we had managed to get a hold on something so toxic.

So positive relationships can be wonderful for teaching us about ourselves; they are incredibly important when it comes to giving kids a happy and secure environment in which to grow up, and they are really fun, especially when you come home late and someone has cooked you something good to eat. But they are ever changing and ever evolving and can either be something you put up with or something you cherish. It's all about choice. I have so much to learn about relationships, but thankfully I do have some wonderful examples around me. But what I do know, or what I am starting to know, is that relationships are very much like gardens; they need tending and loving in order to really be enjoyed. And gnomes are always a bonus. That is the most important lesson.

# 5. Letter to My Boobs: Breastfeeding

*Buongiorno, Funbags!*

*Have you been enjoying your time in solitary confinement? How is it down there in the dark, strapped down and concealed as though you might explode any minute? Fancy some fresh air? A bit of a run around? Maybe a game of rounders? I bet you do. And I'm happy to say that after years of feeling disconnected and distant from you, even though you are right under my nose, I am starting to feel you. In every way.*

*I know you have been starved of love for a long time and I want to address that. Having dutifully produced enough milk to fill the Hoover Dam – resulting in you sometimes resembling two hanging catheter bags – I am starting to, trying to, love you. I most definitely now admire and respect you. I now see that you are gloriously powerful and do not deserve to be shamefully hidden in cavernous beige M&S minimizer bras. You deserve to be adorned in all things beautiful and comfy, and maybe even lace and silk and appreciation. You deserve to be stroked and cupped and tweaked and embraced.*

*I know you feel traumatized by your experience of breastfeeding and I would have understood if you had packed your bags and moved to Uranus after having your sensitive nipples subjected to*

*cracking, bleeding, infection and biting (and not in a fun way).*
*I'm sorry I didn't look after you – I should have done more*
*reading, got more help, protected you from something as simple as*
*a baby at a bad angle.*

*But you have gracefully and proudly performed the life-giving*
*service you were designed for and returned to your former glory*
*(ish) and now it's time you had some fun, and bags of it.*

## Breastfeeding

I've always struggled with my femininity. It doesn't take
much to work out why I'm a bit of a tomboy – I've grown
up with three brothers, I'm good at sport, and I can inhale
Monster Munch faster than any boy I've ever met. I've
also been told I have quite a masculine energy, which I
understand. And whilst there are lots of parts of my
stereotypically 'feminine' self that I am comfortable with,
e.g. my emotional, relational, maternal sides (though
again, just to be clear, these are not exclusively feminine
traits), my boobies have been a part of my anatomy that
I've just done my best to manage, rather than love.

I have such a strange relationship with my boobs. I've
wished they were bigger, I've wished they were smaller,
I've acknowledged them as life-giving and at the same time
found them an inconvenience. Whilst not being gigantically enormous gazongas, they are big enough that when
running for a bus they bounce painfully and awkwardly,

which is annoying. Their size means I can't wear a top without a bra unless I want to look like I'm smuggling two spaniel's ears under my T-shirt and, like dough trying to get through a sieve, they spill unattractively and uncomfortably from little delicate lace bras. Or at least they used to. Because we now, joyfully, live in an era where sexy, affordable bras come in cup sizes above A – thank you, thank you to the person who set that ball rolling.

Why have I never before appreciated their genius and importance? Why have I been so ungrateful for their almost unfathomable brilliance? Why have I been blind to their incredible ability to both produce tailor-made nutrition to a human baby and function as powerful sexual beacons? (That last sentence is definitely enhanced if you make an 'awooga-wooga' noise after reading whilst winding your hips clockwise.)

We women *all* have Wonderboobs. I see other women's boobs and, as an onlooker, understand why they are considered *so* sexy. They are one of the most obvious differences between a woman and a man. Whether big and bouncy or cute and pert, they cheekily protrude from clothes like mischievous meerkats. They are right there, two bonfires of sexuality that refuse to be ignored. They are *gorgeous*. For babies they are their first comfort – they are a pillow, they are intimacy, they give delicious nutrition (yup, I have tried my own breast milk and it tastes like watery vanilla ice cream), they are warm, they provide the opportunity for the mother to enjoy a rush of oxytocin, which is channelled right back into her shiny new chubby cherub, they provide a moment for beautiful, loving eye contact, they are the baby equivalent of a big glass of wine on the sofa with someone you adore. What's not to love?

Whoa, whoa, whoa, hang on one cotton-picking minute. I need to wind my neck in. Whilst I stand by that glorious, hazy vision of boobyliciousness that many people have enjoyed, I am a bit of a fraud. I did not experience that myself. At all.

Breastfeeding for me was neither swift nor smooth. It was more of a laborious roller coaster of fist-clenching pain and was certainly *not* the beautiful booby heaven I've just described. Yes, I'm talking about the most natural thing in the world, the thing our boobs were designed for, and, for me, one of the most hideous experiences of my adult life. (PS stick with this chapter as there is a lesson learned and a happy ending and I really do not want to put anyone off breastfeeding – if it all works and you get good advice, it's flipping amazing for the mum and the kid.)

The experience and the confusion of breastfeeding hit me like a juggernaut hitting a happy but vacant duck sitting in the middle of the road pondering whether to have a little swim or not. It was such a mind-boggling experience that I made a documentary about it for the BBC in 2010 (*Is Breast Best?*). At the time, when the wonderful commissioner suggested this as something to delve into, I did wonder if the topic was going to be too niche to rally any interest. I predicted a flop as floppy as my post-baby boobs. But he was right and I was very wrong. It is one of the highest-rating programmes that I made for BBC Three and had more press coverage and has been the catalyst for more debate than anything else I've ever made. Who knew so many people cared *so* passionately about booby num-nums? (For those that *did* see the programme, you may want to skip this next section as it will feel a little like *Groundhog Day*.)

This was my experience of breastfeeding. When I became pregnant I was anxious about many things. I was concerned about my ability to be a good mum, how it would affect my career, how I would be able to financially support a child, how it would affect my body, how painful the labour would be, whether I could continue to wear trendy hats and Spandex leggings (absolutely yes, was the answer). But I never gave a second thought to breastfeeding. In my mind, it was something that would just happen as naturally and easily as falling off a log. I've got reasonable-sized hooters and, surely, they would do the thing they were made for. I'd lugged them around for long enough and now was the time for them to step up to the breastplate.

I know this sounds ridiculous but I reasoned that, as I wasn't particularly academic but *was* good at sport, and as breastfeeding was a physical activity, I would be OK at this boob-feeding malarky. Yes, because I was good at throwing a javelin I would be good at being milked – totally rational and not at all completely silly. It didn't occur to me to read a book, to prepare, to learn how to do it. It didn't cross my mind that it would require support or equipment or research. I was so arrogant about it that I skipped the antenatal class on breastfeeding so I could work.

So when my wonderful daughter, after being dragged from my being with force and understandably ready for some sustenance, tried to extract some nourishment from my boobs, it was frustratingly difficult for her. And it certainly wasn't a milk-production issue. They were full to the brim. I sometimes wonder if there was a size issue. She seemed so very tiny (although she was a fairly average 6lb 13oz) and my gazongas had exploded into some kind of dairy supernova, so I imagine for her it was a little like trying to have a sip of tea from a garden hose.

Those first few days in hospital are a bit of a blur but I remember quite quickly knowing that she wasn't getting enough nourishment and asking the midwife if she should have a bottle (cue crack of thunder, witch's cackle, werewolf howling, etc.). And because it was clear for all to see that she absolutely wasn't getting enough milk from me, a bottle was produced and she wolfed it down. Over the next four days I had half a dozen different midwives lovingly try to help me get the hang of it. They adjusted her latch, her position, the times of the feeds, the feeding pillow, my posture, my hairstyle (not really but almost) and, in the end, they just scratched their heads and fetched me, with great reluctance and a few cross grumbles, another bottle. Their grumpy reaction completely threw me and was the first stone into the ever expanding pond that is mum-guilt. I just could not understand what the problem was. In my naive state it was simple:

Baby needs milk + boobs not working = bottle good

I couldn't see what part of this simple equation was causing such a negative response, but in my credulous state I didn't realize that I had just entered the complex world of Breastfeeding Politics (cue more witches cackling and ominous music etc.).

I now understand why the midwives had that reaction, but at the time it was extremely annoying that I had tried breastfeeding, observed that it wasn't working and chosen another option, and yet this other option was strangely difficult to procure. This was ludicrous to me. If the hospital stocked formula milk, could it really be so toxic? Thinking about logistics and how busy the ward was, I asked the midwife on duty if she could bring me four or five bottles of milk so that, each time my baby needed feeding, I wouldn't have to bother the overworked nurses. This request was rejected and I was told to carry on trying to breastfeed and only come to the matron's desk to ask for a bottle when it was absolutely necessary. And, because I was in the baby mist where you are so mind-boggled and terrified at having a teeny-tiny fragile human being to take care of, whilst also trying to recover from a major operation to retrieve her from el belly, I said OK and walked the five metres back to my bed (which took approximately fifteen minutes due to the C-section stitches and the catheter).

And so on we went. I tried sitting up in bed with three pillows instead of two, I tried sitting in an upright chair, I tried sitting in a reclining chair, I tried holding her under my armpit like an American football, I tried lying her on my stomach, I tried standing up, I tried lunging . . . (not really, but I would have if it might have worked). Nothing seemed to help and gradually my nipples became very red and very angry.

And that's when I started going into the Bad Booby Place. I was in the baby mist where it's difficult, if not impossible, to make strong, lucid decisions and so I did not take a deep breath and make the conscious and assertive statement that I probably should have. I should have probably stood on my hospital bed with a clanging bell and proclaimed: '*Hear ye! Hear ye! I have tried breastfeeding but it's making both the baby and me very distressed. I have done it for long enough to give her the colostrum milk with all the vital antibodies. I now choose to ensure that she does not wilt with dehydration so I am, without shame, going to give her bottles of formula.*'

But this did not happen. What happened is that I continued this ridiculous charade at home for another three weeks. Every time my baby woke up I would feel utter cold dread. The pain became so bad that I would have to scream into a pillow to stop myself from jumping three feet into the air. Yes, my daughter's first experience of her mummy was a crazed maniac shouting X-rated obscenities into her beautiful, delicate sleepy little face. Good times. Welcome to the world.

My life turned into a two-hour cycle of preparing for breastfeeding (*Gossip Girl* on the laptop, three pillows, pint of water), nappy changing (not mine, although that would have been a brilliant time-saver), intense pain, massaging lotion into my raw nipples, using gauze patches to stop the bleeding, catching a breath, cup of tea . . . and starting all over again. All the cards that were kindly sent to us stating 'Huge Congratulations' seemed like a sick joke.

One of my biggest mistakes was not to voice, to a professional, how extremely painful it was. One day our lovely midwife, Jenny, came to visit and, even though I knew my boobs were in a very bad state, I chose to be a martyr. I was sweating even though I was freezing and had started to get the shakes. But when she asked how I was doing I replied, 'Fine, thanks, breastfeeding is a little painful but I hear that's normal?' After nearly a month of pre- and postnatal hospital care, wonderful husband and mum care, people helping to make the meals and doing the laundry, I just felt that I had used up more than my fair share of moan tokens.

Duuurrr.

What I should have said to her was: 'When I breastfeed I feel like my entire boob is on fire and it's such a painful experience that I cry each time my daughter wakes up in anticipation of the hideous pain.' That would have allowed her to help. But instead, my sweating and shaking progressed over the next twenty-four hours and I rabidly typed ridiculous things into Google, such as 'What do giant red boobs mean?' and 'Help, my boobs are going to explode'.

Thankfully I wasn't the only one typing such ridiculousness into the God that is Google and I came across the wonderful voluntary organization La Leche League. I called their magic twenty-four-hour helpline (I remember feeling so relieved that 'Angry Red Boob Explosion' was common enough to require a twenty-four-hour helpline) and, after hearing my almost uncontrollable sobbing, told me to get into a hot bath and manually massage my boobs to get some of the milk out, thus clearing some of the infection. I tried this – moving very, very slowly so as not to upset the Angry Red Boobs – but they were too painful to touch. So I took a couple of paracetemol, which was like throwing a teeny-tiny pebble into the ocean.

Then one morning I woke up and said to my husband, 'I think I am dying.' (I am a little bit overdramatic.) I had a headache that made my former migraines feel like a tickle, I was sweating profusely all over my body (I'd gone through two towels during the night) and the shakes had become unmanageable. I'd also gone completely grey and was starting to become delirious. So he took me straight to the hospital where I was put into a disused birthing room for five hours whilst they tried to find someone to see me. Unfortunately I'd hit a particularly busy day.

When I was finally seen they immediately took my temperature, put me into a hospital bed and attached me to an IV to flush out my system with antibiotics. One of the funny details I remember was feeling so happy to be in a bed, and such relief that I wasn't actually dying, that I realized I hadn't eaten properly for a couple of days and was duvet-chompingly starving. I asked the nurse for some food and she replied that dinner service had ended. Righto. That really was the cherry on top of a very crappy cake. Thankfully a wonderful woman in the next cubicle heard my pathetic plea and brought me a banana. (Nothing has ever tasted so delicious. I wish I could thank her; that banana meant more than just stomach nourishment.)

Over the next twenty-four hours I returned to the world of the conscious and I learned that I had a very bad case of something called mastitis. Most women, before childbirth, read some sort of breastfeeding article or book and would have known the signs, called the doctor and been prescribed antibiotics before their breasts had fallen off. Not me. I had no idea what this sinister sounding ailment was. Mastitis. It sounds like a James Bond baddie.

On the second day a nurse asked how pumping was going. Huh? Hmm . . . who's pumping what and when exactly? And is this an appropriate chat for a hospital environment? So she carefully explained the exciting world of breast pumping, or 'expressing', or 'milking one-self'. And I listened with much excitement. It was the answer to my prayers. I could avoid having my nipples broken and extract the excess milk from my body *and* give my daughter some lovely milk – *boom town*! Technology has never felt so good.

She took me – slowly, as the breasts were still pretty red and vexed – to 'the pumping room'. Less fun than it sounds. Assuming I was in a fit state to make sense of the expressing machine, she left me to get on with it.

Now let me paint a picture for you. The pumping room was like a stationery cupboard with an office chair and a table with a machine that looked like a scanner. I had been given a clear bag with a long floppy tube, a small bottle and a skin-coloured funnel thingy. And so I sat, tube and bottle in one hand, beige funnel in the other, and tried to A-Team my way into drawing the milk from my boob into the plastic bottle. The machine shouted at me a lot. I think it was trying to tell me that I had inserted the floppy tube into the wrong hole (I had a moment of sympathy for teenage boys) or that I had the funnel upside down or whatever. I kept adjusting positions like some tantric nymphomaniac but to no avail.

Then someone started knocking at the door. I shouted 'Nearly done!' optimistically, until the hormones and the bleeping and the tube flailing about pushed me over the edge and I decided it was OK to have a little cry. And in walked Emily. She had also just had a baby and thus had exploding boobs that needed 'pumping'. She was holding a copy of *Vogue* and, instead of telling me off for hogging the room, she put her arm round me and patiently showed me how to use the machine. And she then gave me her copy of *Vogue* and left me to joyfully and with great relief extract the molten red larva from my exploding volcanoes. I know this is a bit gross, but it was so like squeezing a gigantic spot that is ready to be dealt with that I might have made an orgasm noise. I am still friends with Emily and I will always love her for being kind and giving me *Vogue* to read when I felt very ill and quite scared.

So the IV of antibiotics did its job, both medically and in validating how ill I had felt ('*And they even put me on a drip!*'), and I was given codeine, toast, tea and sleep. Oh, and I watched a whole box set of *The West Wing*. Yeah, I was starting to love mastitis. It took five days for the doctors to feel I was well enough to go home. Because of the risk of hospital infections, Coco hadn't been allowed in with me, and I remember vividly being reunited with her. I got into my brother's car and just held her. It was that kind of breathtaking, intense, overwhelming tidal wave of love where you can't speak or cry or even breathe, but just have to sit still until you come back into your body. It was beautifully bittersweet. We drove home, stopping off at Boots to buy the best expressing machine known to man.

And that's how it went for about five months. I expressed whilst happily and peacefully watching *Gossip Girl*/*The West Wing*/*X Factor*/QVC and then either myself or my husband or my mum would give the milk to her. When I couldn't express enough, we gave her a bottle of formula. And she thrived. I thrived. Finally, free from the terror of having to feed her with raw, bleeding, pus-filled nipples, I started to feel those wonderful new-mum hormones that flood through your body and make your heart explode a little bit.

So, in conclusion, I would deeply and gleefully encourage anyone about to pop with new human life to give

breastfeeding a whirl. Read about it (my absolute favourite guru is the boob goddess Clare Byam-Cook – I tried
her method with my son and actually cracked it), watch
videos about it (again, Clare's DVDs are fab but there are
so many on YouTube) and ask as many other mums as
possible for advice.

It is so worth having a really good go, doing some research
and asking for help. It is just lovely for everyone if it works
and it's free – hello, thank you. BUT for all the *love* in the
world, PLEASE, please, if you find that it's really painful, my
best, most loving advice would be to bite your lip for two or
three days until your baby has taken in your amazing antibodies in the form of the colostrum milk, and then look at other
options. Because there *are* other options. And ploughing on
like a real trooper because you feel that everyone around you
would judge you for mix-feeding or bottle-feeding, whilst you
are bleeding and cracking and crying into a pillow IS NOT
AN OPTION. It doesn't even have to be as silly and dramatic
as my experience. It can be half, less than half, as bad and still
be awful. Please don't let my insane pain be in vain.

In *Is Breast Best?* (yup, you can imagine how that title
went down . . .) I investigated the reaction I had faced in
the hospital and subsequent remarks I had been treated
to when feeding Coco with a bottle. I realized that I felt
shame each time someone looked over at us. It was probably due to a mixture of the hospital reaction and something that was already in me and I think I started to join
the dots. If breast really *is* best, as the slogan goes, and

my baby *isn't* getting that, what did that make *me*? Of course the slogan 'Breast is Best but Bottle Will Do if You're Screaming into the Pillow' is less catchy. But for all of the statement's clever, memorable alliteration, it made me feel like a rubbish mum. It made me feel like a mum who obviously didn't mind giving her kid something deeply unhealthy. And that felt awful. As a new mum I was extremely vulnerable to criticism – because I had no idea what I was doing. I knew I was doing my best but that didn't seem good enough. I knew that my system of giving my baby expressed milk in a bottle worked for us, but the looks I was given (from people who assumed I was giving formula milk) and the articles I read to prepare for the programme shocked me. It seemed that everyone had an opinion. That's when I encountered the Breastfeeding Mafia.

'Breastfeeding Mafia' is a derogatory name for a group of women who are simply passionate about breastfeeding. But there are extremists, as there are in every group, and in this case they take the form of women who won't even entertain the possibility of a microscopically tiny benefit of using a bottle.

I travelled down to Brighton one sunny day to meet a self-confessed group of breastfeeding evangelists for tea, cake and some full-on public breastfeeding. Having never really seen breastfeeding in public, especially not with children over fifteen months old and definitely never without any cover, I felt a great deal of love for this amazing group of women who believed that it wasn't necessary to hide in the shadows when doing something as natural and necessary as feeding their baby. At the time I didn't feel brave enough to do the same, and I now *know*, having attempted to feed my son Bear in a similarly open way, that I'm not – it's strangely scarier than it might seem. Anyway, at that point I agreed wholeheartedly with their message and loved their passion – I felt solidarity with the group and wondered why some people reacted so negatively towards them.

We then moved on to the subject of bottles. I tried to hide my 'What the fuck?!' face when they told me that there was never, *ever* a time when it was OK to use formula. (Now I know better than to dive into this debate head first without a disclaimer: this is an extremely complicated subject. It goes as far as including conspiracy theories regarding the large formula companies, but I am going to steer well clear of that arena. I can only speak from my personal experience and try to be as honest as possible.) What *I* experienced was distress at not being able to feed my baby and acute pain. And, until I had discovered the joys of expressing my own milk, a bottle of formula was as welcome as rain after a drought. And I could see that my baby was fed and fine. And my daughter is still fine. She very rarely gets ill and is as strong as an ox. Our bond is wonderful.

So I would say, based on my experience, that the blanket scaremongering and guilt-hustling put on new mums using bottles is absolutely ludicrous. *Of course* booby-feeding is incredible and has wonderful health benefits, for both the mum and the baby, and is to be encouraged. But I feel that the beauty and importance of that message has also picked up the unfortunate and unnecessary subtext of '*Mothers who use bottles are bad mothers who don't really care.*'

Even if a mum *has* chosen to bottle-feed her baby without trying to breastfeed, she has her reasons. When making the programme, I spoke to some young mums who had chosen, consciously, to bypass breastfeeding altogether. And they had their, very valid, reasons. In their circle, if you breastfed, you would be called a slag. And you would be bullied. And neither their grandmothers nor their mums had breastfed. In their community it was not something *anyone* did. And so these young girls, already feeling pretty vulnerable and vilified by society, had chosen bottles and formula. To me that is more than understandable. And wow, as very young mums, with everything else they have to cope with, surely the last thing anyone would want is for them to then carry the guilt of using a bottle. Seriously? I'm not saying that they shouldn't receive the same education about the benefits of breastfeeding as other mums, or that they shouldn't have the same help and support if they choose to try it, but I do think that if, after all of that, they still decide to use a bottle, their decision should be accepted and understood without being made to feel guilty with lashings of patronizing judgement.

I know other mums who, because of past trauma, chose to immediately bottle-feed. And because of the personal nature of their experience, they did not share this with medical staff or other mums they encountered on a day-to-day basis. But, even with perfectly understandable reasons to go straight for the bottle, they had to deal with judgemental looks and comments. What a lovely start to being a parent. Even showing a single frame of a baby being fed by a bottle in the opening credits of the programme caused a lot of anger.

So I repeat this message loud and clear, so that at least if I get abuse it will be for something I truly believe and not because of a misunderstanding:

- Yes, breastfeeding is absolutely the best for the mum and for the baby.
- Yes, we should be spreading the word about how wonderful and natural it is to those that don't yet know.
- Yes, we should be encouraging mums to learn how to breastfeed in a non-screaming-into-the-pillow way.
- Yes, we should be encouraging people to donate to milk banks to give mums who don't produce enough breast milk, or for other reasons do not want to breastfeed, other options and, of course, to ensure that babies in intensive care have more than enough to go round. But the above messages should also come with a proviso: 'Give it your best shot but don't suffer in

silence as there are other, perfectly good, options.' This proviso should be heard loud and clear.

- And no, we should not be telling mothers that it will affect the bond with their child when that is, in my experience, incorrect, inconclusive and has caused utterly pointless guilt and anxiety for many new mums.
- Finally, no, we should never give a new mum who has chosen to bottle-feed, for her own reasons, dirty looks in cafés. Ever.

OK, I am bracing myself for the backlash but that's what long runs and friends are for.

So, with all this new knowledge of boobs, machines, lotions and helplines, when my second child Bear popped out I felt like a commando about to go into battle. And when I could tell that the same problem was happening, I immediately called upon the expert help of the breastfeeding guru Clare Byam-Cook to come and have a gander. (I promise she does not sponsor me; I just believe her to be magic.) She gave me some sage advice – which she has been deeply criticized for – but which made perfect sense to me. It went along the lines of: '*Give breastfeeding a go; it's definitely better for the baby and the mum, but if it's causing distress then try mix-feeding, or expressing or bottle-feeding. Essentially your baby will be fine, but screaming into your arm at 5 a.m. isn't right.*' Clare also says "If *neither* the baby *nor* a breast pump can get enough milk out of *your* breasts, it's better to supplement with formula than to have an unhappy, hungry and underweight baby". Formula milk is *not* liquid poison.

So that's what I did. When breastfeeding started making me want to recite Eminem's raps, I decided to both boob-feed and express and use formula. And lo and behold, because I was giving them a break, my boobs never became horrendously painful so I was able to continue breastfeeding for longer. I even got into that lovely place where I looked forward to feeding time. About a month after giving birth, my boobs had calmed down and they became soft enough for Bear to get a comfortable latch fairly easily. It was beautifully cosy. And for a while I could see why some women are so evangelical about it, almost to the point of aggression – because when it works, it's wonderful, and essentially their motive is positive and loving because it comes from their desire for other women and babies to enjoy that experience.

I'm glad I persevered the second time, even if it's just to say with experience that sometimes the bottle isn't evil. For me and other women, it's a breathing space for their boobs to recover, which can, in turn, give them enough strength to carry on trying to breastfeed for longer.

OK, I'll see you on Twitter for what I imagine will be a colourful response. (*Brace! Brace!*)

# 6. Letter to My Belly: Diets, Pregnancy

*Dear Belly,*

*Can I call you that? I really hate the word 'stomach'; it sounds like an STD. But 'tummy' makes me think of a Care Bear and 'midriff' brings me out in hives. And sorry for diving right in there but I'm going to put my cards on the table and say I have spent most of my life just not really liking you. I'm not talking about the actual stomach organ – that is actually very useful and I need that in order to deal with the weekly Friday-night nacho assault. I'm addressing that part of my anatomy between my boobs and my fanny. I'm talking to that bit that requires an elasticated waistband after Christmas lunch (or nachos). I'm dealing with that bit we're told needs to be as flat as a pancake, which is ironic as pancakes are most definitely not on the menu if you want a flat-pancake stomach. Yeah, belly area, I'm talking to you.*

*In fact, you have really pissed me off. Why do you need to be flat? Why can't you be beautiful and slightly rounded? Why can't it be gorgeous and sexy and womanly for you to be curved? (Oh, it can, it's just not at all reflected in our media.)*

*Growing up, as someone who had two beady eyes on the media, I have tried to behave and do my stomach exercises and not eat pasta after 6 p.m. (mostly unsuccessfully) but you refused to submit to my will. Why do other girls seem to effortlessly work a midriff so taut that you could bounce a ping-pong ball off it? In a world where a woman's value seems to be connected to how she looks in a bandage dress, why won't you just stop protruding like you've got something to say? Do you have something to say? Well, sodding spit it out and then we can all get on with our lives.*

*Sorry. You don't deserve that rant. Because, recently, our relationship has turned a corner and things have changed. I'm now thirty-four and the womb that nestles inside you has beautifully, magically produced two human beings. Thank you from the depths of my heart. But, frustratingly, even though you have carried out this most miraculous of feats, old habits die hard and I still sometimes revert to my sixteen-year-old self who wants to wear a trendy cut-out swimming costume without looking like jelly trying to escape from a string bag. I both revere you and despair of you.*

*But, even though my vain teenage self still wails sometimes, the glory of getting older is that that voice does start to fade. And marvelling at your ability to grow a baby has started to override any frustration that your preferred status is rotund. I salute myself that I am now wise enough to realize that producing human life might be slightly more important than being able to wear crop tops. Yeah, hardly Germaine Greer, but we're getting there.*

## Diets

Like working out how old a tree is by how many rings it has, I think you could probably age a woman by the diets she has tried. Or maybe that's just me. Because, you name it, I have tried it. You know those annoying online adverts that say 'Click Here for Miracle Weight Loss – I Lost 7lbs by Eating Only Cheese'? I think most people just chortle at how ridiculous they are and wonder what kind of mug clicks on them. Well, I was that mug. They were like catnip. And every magazine article that promised the same miracle solution had the same effect.

My first diet was after I realized that I was noticeably rounder than my friends who, much to my surprise, seemed to remain standing in a strong wind. So, armed with little to no information about nutrition (as is right for a sixteen-year old) I set about trying to correct the 'problem'. I say 'problem' because really I should have left myself alone. It wasn't a 'problem'; it was just my body growing up. But, because of my meddling, I made it a real problem, which then took me a further sixteen years to fix. Nice one, Chesa.

A little like 'my first keyboard' or 'my first bicycle', 'my first diet' was amateur. My chosen method was to delegate the problem to my mother. I know what you're thinking. *That is a recipe for trouble.* And you would be right.

One day, when I was sixteen and about to go on holiday to France with some girlfriends, my lovely mother decided to take me on a shopping trip to buy a swimming costume at a department store. How wonderful. How bonding. Sadly, but perhaps predictably, this ended with me standing half naked in the changing rooms silently crying at how hideous my body was as I grabbed my wobbly tummy and looked forlornly at the huge cardboard cut-out of a thin, tanned, taut woman flouncing about in a white cut-out swimming costume that was propped up next to the mirror. It was so depressing and such a formative moment that, nearly two decades later, I can still vividly remember what she looked like. (An aside: what kind of sadistic shop would put that in a changing room?!)

So I looked at Cardboard Cut-out Girl and I looked at me. There I was, standing like a piece of (in my eyes) sad, pale, uncooked pastry under the changing-room lights, spilling out of my Lycra cage of pain and inwardly wailing, *Why oh why don't I look like her?* Slightly dramatic I know but at sixteen that was my default setting. I'm ashamed to admit in that moment any sense of perspective of how lucky I was to be healthy and from a happy family with enough money to go on holiday in the first place was completely and utterly lost on me. But as I said, I was sixteen.

It was after this tiny meltdown that I asked my mum to help me. And because she loves me she agreed to assist in my mission (when she should have really run away screaming). So we made an agreement that she would make me healthy food and discourage me from second helpings. Gosh, it seemed like such a good idea at the time, like having a personal chef. But the problem was that, in practice, I loathed it. Instead of feeling grateful that she didn't offer me a second helping of her manna-from-heaven bread-and-butter pudding, but *did* offer it to my brothers and their girlfriends, I felt awful. And instead of telling her that our agreement wasn't having the desired effect and was making me feel very pants, I just got angry. And then a little bit angrier. And then I turned into A Teenager. And, having been pretty easy-going, I started to behave like A Big Bitch. I expressed my dissatisfaction at my physical appearance and my anger at my mother's insinuation that I was fat (yup, that's how I interpreted her attempts to help me) by being cold and mean and cross. And because this chapter is about my stomach and not about me being a bitch I'll close this diet story by saying that my mum gladly gave up her role as my private dietician and we hugged and made up.

My next few attempts at changing my body shape were sometimes on the right track but were mostly as mad as a March hare. By this time I was in sixth form and, because we were over sixteen and were legally allowed to have sex and become mothers, the school deemed it acceptable for us to also be allowed into the sports facilities in the morning. So I took this new freedom and I ran with it. Literally. I decided that, because I loved sport, this was my ticket to metamorphosing into the bronzed cardboard goddess in the cut-out swimming costume.

Every morning I would wake up at 5.30 a.m., drag myself out of bed, run to the gym, work out for forty minutes or swim (I hate swimming), run back to the boarding house, shower, drink coffee, eat breakfast and then get ready for the walk to school at 8.15 a.m. At first this was excruciatingly painful (and at the end of every day I felt like I deserved a medal) but quickly I became used to the dark early mornings, the frosty cold and the red nose. This could have potentially become quite a reasonable solution to becoming healthier and slimmer but because it was motivated by self-loathing, not self-love, it was miserable. I took it to the extreme and my nutritional awareness was slim to none, thus placing it at *numero due* on the list of failed diets.

Thanks to the relentless early mornings, the extensive exercise (I was also playing sport twice a week and at the weekends) and the long days at school preparing for A levels, I was exhausted and therefore ate three times my body weight in toast and jam and chocolate buttons and brownies and chips and anything I could get my munchy mitts on. It took perhaps a month of this routine to clock on to the fact that, despite running around like a headless muppet and doing more exercise than most Olympic athletes, I had actually put weight *on* and needed a pair of pliers to do up my jeans. Plus I was really, really tired and had blisters.

So I decided that perhaps waking up at 5.30 a.m. and eating lots of toast was not the miracle solution. Time for a different approach. By this time I was eighteen and my A levels were approaching fast. Thanks to my glorious history of art teacher I was doing OK and was generally having a great time at school feeding my brain with excellent things. Which is why my next attempt at becoming the Cardboard Cut-out Girl was so ridiculous.

I thought, *Well, if avoiding second helpings doesn't work and if lots of exercise isn't the answer, then maybe I need to just stop eating.* Or just eat carrots. Or just a brown roll for lunch. Or pears, because another girl was doing that (this is the infection of eating problems) and it seemed to be working for her. Yeah. All of those happened. At one point my house mistress (a kind of surrogate mum whilst you're at boarding school) called me into her office to discuss my obscene consumption of carrots. She was concerned that I would gradually turn orange (which is possible) and that perhaps I should include the other food groups in my diet. And of course because I was still doing long days at school and playing sport during the week my fuel gauge was constantly at empty. So yes I did lose some weight but I also turned grey and boring and grumpy and tired and crappy. I was, in fact, so crappy that my lovely friends staged an intervention.

I remember it vividly. It was 9 p.m. and instead of joining the girls in the corridor for a feast of tea, toast and hilarious sex/poo/boy chat, I had once again tucked myself up in bed because I was exhausted. And I will forever be pathetically grateful to my friends because they caught me before my eating insanity potentially turned into something serious and life-changing – and not in a good way. In no uncertain terms they told me that I wasn't being a good friend, that I was boring, that they missed me, that I was an idiot for letting my grades slip because I was too tired to do my coursework and that grey didn't suit me. They were kind but extremely firm. Thank God. It was done with love and protection and it woke me up.

The thing that particularly bothered me was that I was being a crap friend. I knew I was being boring because I was boring myself. In order to find the willpower to only eat a single bread roll for an entire day, it took such a *mammoth* amount of self-discipline and mental energy that I had become completely obsessed with achieving it. Essentially I had become *entirely* self-obsessed and quite depressed. I didn't have any energy or brain-space for my friends, for their needs or their company. They were right – I *was* being a horribly rubbish friend. So I stopped being a plonker and started eating again. My skin turned pink and my poo jokes got better and I laughed and skipped and felt human again. And I didn't eat carrots for a long time.

Then I left school and, cringe, went travelling. Yes, bead necklace, baggy tie-up Thai trousers and trekking sandals. Oh, I could not have been more of a stereotype if I had tried. I loved every minute of it. I even 'found myself'. During this wonderful time swimming in warm blue seas and climbing mountains and meeting new people from countries I couldn't even spell and staying in ant-infested huts and sleeping on the floor of buses and dancing to rave music whilst covered in UV paint and exploring caves and jumping into lagoons and seeing a year's worth of actual live sunsets (they look just how they do on Instagram) and eating noodle soup and drinking whisky out of a little red bucket and riding motorbikes without a licence and getting very sunburnt, I forgot about wanting to be slim and just lapped up every minute of every day of the incredible freedom and adventure. And because of irony or sod's law or both, I lost some weight and became a healthy size and could zip up my trousers without even wincing. I should have learned from this experience that happy exercise and happy eating was quite a good combo for feeling healthy and maintaining a good weight, but I didn't. Because I am a numpty.

I came back from this wondrous experience and showed my beads and tan to anyone and everyone, realized that I looked like a twat wearing my Thai fisherman's trousers in the middle of London, got a haircut, bought some deodorant and went to university. The first year, just speaking bodily, was fantastic. I felt great. I had tons of energy. I was fit and strong and comfortable in my own skin. I enjoyed getting dressed and shopping and ate and drank whatever I wanted. And this is where I became unstuck. I didn't look after my new body. I think, somewhere deep down, I wondered if I could now be like other girls and just eat whatever I wanted (at the time I was totally unaware that nearly all people have to think about what they eat – it's very personal and not something everyone talks about).

Because I was eating rubbish by the bath-load (I can be a touch gluttonous) but wasn't climbing mountains or dancing until dawn every day, and was instead getting the bus, sitting in a lecture hall for six hours, mooching around at my friends' flats, sitting on the bus again and then going to bed, my fit and comfortable body started to disappear.

And, vexingly, rather than being relaxed about it and deciding to shift my eating and exercise habits back to the healthy, happy status of the previous year, I had a big freak-out and decided to hit the gym hard and try to find a miracle diet cure. Oh God, I can feel as I write this that my face has set into a pained expression of sad, exasperated frustration because I am remembering just how awful this period was and each memory is more pathetic and embarrassing than the next. The people sitting around me in this café must think I'm reading a really sad email. I hope I don't spontaneously burst into tears and have to tell them that I'm actually fine, I'm just remembering eating fistfuls of ham in a car park. Jeeezzz.

I got myself into such a terrible cycle of dieting and self-loathing that it pains me to think about what a waste of time and money it was when I could have been laughing and learning and kissing and frolicking and dancing and doing all the things you should be doing at university – all of which I *did* do, but the joy I felt doing them was compromised by thinking about how I was going to achieve the holy grail of 'thinness'.

I haven't mentioned that word yet: 'thin.' That tiny word is one of my least favourite in the English language. It has stolen so much of my brain-time and happiness that if I met it in the street I would put it in a headlock and poke its eyes. Because from my mid-teens I wanted to be thin – desperately. Maybe it was all of those nineties pictures of heroin-chic models standing around in their pants with bones jutting out, looking a bit depressed and ever so slightly like Gollum but with better eyebrows and a spot of bronzer. Maybe it was the actresses and singers and movie stars that seemed to exist by photosynthesizing. I don't know.

However it came about, I wanted to be really, really thin. And tall. And ethereal and mysterious – just like those models in the magazines that hover about in chiffon and recline on big rocks in the desert with lots of smoky eye make-up and sometimes a Dalmatian near by for effect. Which, for a loud, sporty, short, extrovert girl, was never going to happen. I *now* know that I will never, ever, be the tall girl reclining on the rock in chiffon – and because I am thirty-four I have made peace with that and have also realized that being ethereal and mysterious and very, very thin (unless it's natural) often results in needing to smoke a lot, possibly eat loo paper (a real thing) and being fantastically self-obsessed and thus extremely boring. But at the time I was blinded by the idea that this was the ideal woman and I wanted to look like her.

So, back to university dietary hideousness. At the end of my second year, I experienced my first bout of heartbreak, which, I learned, is Kryptonite for a woman's bottom. Thankfully my friend Polly helped nurse me back to health by cooking me delicious, healthy suppers (mostly salmon and broccoli, which neither of us can now eat) and encouraging me to go for the occasional Fun Run with her. Polly is so brilliant that she simply re-branded exercise – *'Hey, let's go and be silly at the park and run about and laugh and chase each other and it will be really fun!'* – and therefore she turned physical movement from a painful chore into a joy.

And, once again, I *should* have continued on this excellent path because it was working and was healthy and non-insane. But did I? No, no, no. Instead I once again started to seek out the quick-fix cure that would miraculously turn me into a thin six-foot goddess with legs long enough to plait. And this leads me on to my next cycle of doom: laxatives.

This perhaps wins the prize for the most horrible, dangerous attempt at losing weight and I tell it with a heavy heart at the realization that I was desperate enough to even think about it. I don't know where I got the idea and I certainly didn't do any research into how dangerous it was, I just did it. I won't go into the gory details, as we all know what happens when you take laxatives, but as you can imagine it was pretty grim. And, because it was something my body got used to, I had to take more and more to get the same effect. Yes, it eventually worked but not in the way I had imagined. Because I was taking so many pills, I developed terrible stomach pains that were sometimes so bad I could barely stand and most certainly couldn't eat. Which *of course* results in weight loss, but also makes leaving the house tricky, spending time with friends almost impossible and doing anything fun at all, including reading or writing (fairly useful whilst at university), and sometimes breathing, a challenge. Super fun.

Then I started getting headaches. Then weird pains in my legs. And then, in a rare moment of lucidity, I staged an intervention on myself and stopped taking them because whilst I did want to be thin I didn't want to be dead. It took a while for my body to recover from this toxic assault but I am so grateful that I don't seem to have done any irreversible damage. The only thing that was hurt was my pride at being such a massive twonk.

You would think at that point, after such an unpleasant experience, I would try something more sustainable and healthy. You've guessed it – No I Didn't! Next came the Atkins Diet. Most people know that this diet involves eating only protein, but what they may not know is how much harder this is in practice than on paper. And, more than any other diet, it taught me that cutting out entire food groups, for me, is nuts, miserable, impossible to sustain and plays havoc with my precious, delicate metabolism and, just as importantly, my mental state. Like all of these cray-cray diets, it works for a little bit, which is why there are hundreds of forums expressing the miraculous properties of these lotions/potions/notions, but then you turn into an actual cray-cray person.

And, because you are – I was – wearing rose-tinted/desperate goggles, I ignored any online comments containing negative reports, but instead only read about how lives had been changed and bodies transformed by eating only cheese and yoghurt and steak and eggs and mayonnaise. *Wow!* It was too good to be true! (It *was* too good to be true.) I did this diet with my flatmate and, whilst the diet itself remained horrible, it felt good to have a comrade rather than doing it in a little secret world of embarrassment. At least when it became particularly absurd we could laugh about it together. I have some fond(ish) memories of the two of us standing in our underwear like something out of *Withnail and I* staring into the fridge and acknowledging the insanity that it only contained cottage cheese, sliced ham and beef. It was a very bonding experience. Sharing this bonkers part of my life made me feel very vulnerable and I love knowing that someone else felt this way too. I have no doubt that we will still laugh about it when we are old and wrinkly.

So we did this diet for a few months, lost some weight, put it back on, lost it again and put it back on. And, as I'd experienced with the Bread Roll Diet, the Atkins Diet also turned you grey. Even my eyes turned a pallid, lacklustre beige. Eventually we came to the realization that we both wanted to stop eating packets of ham as a snack and wanted to eat in normal restaurants and enjoy being human again. Having eggs for breakfast, chicken for lunch and beef for supper sounds great but do that for more than a week and it becomes gag-tastic. When you start fantasizing about an apple you know something isn't right.

As a side note, I have known people that have really loved this diet as a way to kick-start some weight loss, but even in this case it is most certainly not something that is healthy to do for more than a few weeks.

By the time I left university I had experimented with the cayenne-pepper diet, the children's-purée diet, the eat-only-from-a-small-plate diet, the chew-100-times diet, the detox-supplement-and-water-only diet, the juice-only diet, the coffee-and-cold-bath diet and the Dukan Diet. (The Dukan is mildly better than the Atkins in that it won't turn your arteries into solid clogged lard pipes, but it doesn't teach you about portion control or when/how to eat happily, so you will either remain in the misery of only being able to eat ham *or* you will crack and put the weight back on, plus a few pounds.)

Eventually, so slowly that you'd be justified in thinking I had jam for brains, I started to realize that *perhaps* these miracle diets *didn't* work and perhaps someone was making a lot of money each time I bought into their diet bars/shakes/books/pills. Essentially they were making money from my pitiful desperation to be something I was never going to be. And I realized that *maybe* the answer had been staring me in the face all this time and *maybe* my mother was right (don't you hate it when that happens?) – in other words, moderation was the key. BORING! However, I reluctantly accepted that the only thing more boring was taking Miracle Hot Chilli capsules, wanting to be sick on a daily basis and *still* not losing the promised weight for more than a few days.

With nothing left, I decided to give 'eating normally' a try. And lo and behold, it worked. It was frustratingly slow but it produced results. And I wasn't behaving like a crazy ham-obsessed moron *or* eating from a tiny child's plate like a complete idiot *or* consuming only green gunk that made my tongue furry and my poo smell like cut grass (quite nice, actually). I started to behave and feel like a 'normal' person (if there is such a thing). I realized that, as a short woman, my body didn't need that much food so, as someone who loves food, I needed to work out how best to use my food tokens. And, as someone who loves exercise, I should make sure the exercise I did always made me feel happy and strong and fit, but not do so much that it made me ravenous and exhausted and depressed and wanting to eat chocolate at 2 a.m.

So, after the highs and lows and carrots and pills, I finally found a happy place. And here is the secret to this happy place. Are you ready? It's going to make me millions. Buckle up, here we go.

## The One-Size-Does-Not-Fit-All Diet

Wow, can't you hear the megabucks pouring into my bank? Can't you see the headlines and the star status and the magazine covers and the supermodel clients and the six-figure book deal?

Yes, after my dietary odyssey, I have realized that we are all different and one size does not fit all. If there were a billion people on the planet then there should be a billion different diets. We all need different amounts of sleep, sex and shopping, we all have the capacity for different intensities of emotion, workload and fun, we all have different food, art and music preferences, and I truly believe the same can be applied to what and when and how our bodies want to be fed. The idea that we should all eat in the same way is crackers.

For example, I think it's a shame that so many children are taught to finish everything on their plate, and then spend their twenties learning how to stop eating when they are full. I remember vividly sitting in the school hall with the dreaded (well, for me anyway) fish pie and visibly gagging as the teacher made me finish it. It took me two decades to eat fish again; even the smell made me feel sick. Every mealtime was an experiment in precisely determining how much you needed to eat – take too little and you'd be hungry for the rest of the day, take too much and you'd be forced to push through your pain barrier until your plate was clean. The habit is so ingrained in me that when my children's friends come for supper I sometimes automatically congratulate them on their 'nice clean plates'. Again, crackers.

In the same vein, the received wisdom, vehemently promoted as though it is scientific gospel, is that breakfast is the most important meal of the day and therefore should never be skipped. It took me a long time to realize that how you start your day *is* important but it isn't about eating a lot, but rather making sure that you make the best choice for you. And, for *my* body, I've learned that eating a lot, or often anything at all, first thing in the morning makes me sluggish and sometimes a bit nauseous. And generally eating breakfast just makes me hungrier at lunchtime. For a lot of my friends not eating breakfast turns them into a spaced-out rage-zombie. I was talking to my mum about this the other day and she reminded me about our daily breakfast tussle whilst I was at primary school. I was so adamant that I didn't want to eat anything that I became a master at hiding toast in different nooks in the house. I wonder whether I knew instinctively at that age that my body didn't want feeding until later in the day. Or it might have been because I was a pain in the arse. But despite this, as a mother now, even knowing that everybody is different, I could never send my daughter to school on an empty stomach. Yup, total hypocrite.

It's taken me a long time to work out that my body functions best when I eat very lightly during the day and do my main feeding after 5 p.m. – a little like a vampire. As someone who adores cooking and eating out with friends in the evening, it seems to be a good balance. And on the whole, if I'm also exercising, it seems to work. It means I can go to a restaurant and choose something because my stomach requests it, rather than the default option of the sodding Caesar salad. It's liberating.

# Post-Preggers Weight

I know that for some women it just falls off, but that certainly isn't me. After I gave birth I had two options: work my tits off to get back to my pre-baby weight, or buy an entire new wardrobe of clothes. And it was encouraging to hang out with my friends who are mums who felt the same. The myth that it comes off on its own is just that, a myth – for me at least. Two years after my son was born and, whilst I still have a way to go, I am gradually getting my pre-preg fitness back.

I know it's not cool to be so open about how these things are worked out – I know that it's much cooler to say the usual 'I just don't really think about it', but I have the suspicion that, for most of us, we *do* have to think about it. Sometimes in interviews I get asked if I have any health secrets and I always say that it's exercise and involves being really thoughtful about what I eat. Before I realized that I wasn't the kind of woman whose weight just 'fell off', I used to stare at girls eating burgers and lasagne and shepherd's pie and BLTs and wonder How the France they managed to eat those things whilst still being slim, whilst I was stuck having a crappy salad. As I poked my steamed vegetables with frustrated contempt I wondered whether perhaps these girls were super-dooper lucky or had ringworm. I would then go home and eat a low-fat yoghurt, an apple, a low-fat hot chocolate, another apple, a few Ryvita and maybe another apple – and perhaps another Ryvita with Ultra-Light-Tastes-Like-Body-Lotion cream cheese, if I was *really* treating myself.

But I now know, and wish I had known earlier, that because the things I ate were low fat, they were completely unsatisfying and I would therefore keep grazing as my body desperately searched for something containing nutrition. I think on a cellular level I was probably starving. The end result was that I was consuming *more* calories than if I had just eaten something delicious and satisfying in the first place.

And I now know, and wish I had known earlier, that because my friend who tucked into lasagne and normal foods had chosen something healthy and real, and had eaten a normal portion and had *enjoyed* her food, she was satisfied – and therefore didn't spend the rest of the night snacking. And *because* she was eating delicious, nutritious food, she didn't feel starved or that food was rationed, so the temptation to pick or snack was reduced and she enjoyed the feeling of waiting until her next satisfying meal before eating again. The whole cycle was healthy and happy. It was, in fact, *not unfair at all* but simple physics, with a side order of psychology. She was eating *fewer* calories than me and enjoying her food more.

And I now know, and wish I had known earlier, that it doesn't matter if I am eating *low-fat* cereal – if I eat six bowls, then I might as well have had something really tasty rather than something that tastes like cat litter. A revelation. I now know that 'fat' isn't bad; depending on which kind and how much you have, it's quite the opposite. An avocado is very fatty but it tastes amazing and is incredibly satisfying and sends fantastically effective signals to your brain that tell your body it's had enough. Bonza. Plus it's 'good fat' and won't clog your arteries like animal lard. Avocado, nuts and oily fish all have the magic effect of making me feel fuller and faster (I sound like an M&S advert) – they're proper super-foods and they taste about three million times better than a piece of cardboard, aka a diet cracker.

And I now know, and wish I had known earlier, that low-fat yoghurts might be 'fat-free' but they are in fact chock-a-block full of sugar, which is *technically* non-fat, but once inside us creates more fat. So, if sugar turns to fat in the body, the claim that they are 'low-fat' is surely false advertising. Because, yes, on the shelf they don't contain fat, but as soon as we pop it into our bodies it turns into fat. I know it's a technicality but surely, with a country struggling to cope with the rising number of obese people, it's a fairly important point to note on a label?

In any case, after a day of eating dietary foods with bugger all in them other than synthetic flavours, sugar, artificial thickeners and sweeteners, my body rebels with the ferocity of a tiger attacking a gazelle and suddenly I find myself eating fistfuls of crap at the wrong time of night. And this is because it is hungry on a cellular level. Yes, I might have put 'food' into my mouth but it did not have enough nutrition. So then my survival mechanism kicks in and I raid the fridge at 11.30 p.m. It's bonkers, it's unpleasant and it prevents you from enjoying the wonderful social joy of proper food. I hate that I did this and was robbed of eating in a happy, non-embarrassing way.

What I now know, and wish I had known earlier, is that laughing with friends over a beautiful bowl of pasta and a big glass of wine is so much happier than standing on your own in front of the fridge in your PJs shovelling bread and chocolate spread into your mouth at binge-o'clock. Sharing food, eating together, trying new restaurants and cooking new recipes is one of the great joys of my life. I would love to live in a world where there was no need for *anyone* to spend *any* hard-earned money on sugar-packed, low-fat, nutritionally void 'food' because everyone was enjoying proper wholefood and feeling great about it.

I love the recent campaign #fitnotthin; it's absolutely the message we should be encouraging. Fit comes in all shapes and sizes; fit helps you to enjoy your body and life; fit gives you energy and is obtainable. This message is positive, healthy and achievable. I wish I had caught on to this message earlier, but better late than never. I have finally stopped (well, started to stop) pining for a body that I'll never, ever have – therefore creating only unhappiness and frustration – and started to be grateful for and look after the one I've got. I know this doesn't sound trumpet-worthy, but I also know that there are so, so many girls and women out there who will understand that that is a seismic shift.

## Pregnancy

Hard to believe, but there is a force at work that is *even* more powerful than that cardboard-cut-out swimming-costume girl. It's being up the duff. Now that I am a mum I have a whole new appreciation of the stupendous flexibility of the belly. As I sit here writing this, my stomach is sitting only inches away quietly and gracefully(ish) recovering from baby *numero due*. It's taken quite a beating and being stretched to within an inch of its life without popping is quite impressive. And it all started in a loo in a shopping centre . . .

In 2008 I had my first out-of-body experience. I was working at the BBC on a holiday programme for kids where the children make all the decisions and inevitably choose activities, such as paragliding, that scare the bejesus out of their parents. It was a hoot and I loved every minute of it. I was also about to go on my first big filming trip abroad as a trainee assistant producer and it felt like a huge and exciting milestone in my career.

And, on an otherwise unremarkable day, I popped into the local shopping centre, Westfield, for some lunch. And as I mooched along thinking about which type of deliciousness to put into my pie-hole, I noticed that my boobs felt very bulbous. Hmmm, interesting. My weight felt the same and my bra was an old beige minimizer from M&S . . . what possible reason could there be for having big bazookas today? And then the realization started creeping in, like a cloud of smog descending over Beijing, that my period was perhaps slightly tardy . . . Hmmm, interesting. But no, no, no, I couldn't be . . . I couldn't possibly be . . . I had a coil. Which meant that, um, I was not . . .

I couldn't be . . .

I must not be . . .

And so, laughing at the ridiculousness of it, I bought a pregnancy test in Superdrug and went to wee on a stick. I had never done this before and, as a big fan of new experiences, thought that perhaps it might be, at the very least, an interesting or a funny story to tell the Ladies. I was so convinced that this was a ridiculous thing to do that I didn't even take my headphones out and continued to bop along to Usher. And so I did the deed and peed on the stick. And I waited.

And then I fell off a cliff.

My entire being fell off a cliff. Out of my body and off a cliff.

Because I was pregnant.

I was pregnant.

I was fucking pregnant.

And my being kept on falling. Further and further away from my body until I thought I was going to pass out.

I know this sounds absurdly overdramatic, but at the time it felt like a tornado had blown away the delicate house of cards I had painstakingly and passionately been building and I felt the huge reality of it descend in one small moment. You know how some things take a while to sink in? Well, this didn't. This was like being hit by an anvil.

For the past few years I had worked every minute of every day to climb slowly up the production ladder – desperate and excited and hungry to become a director. And this little blue line put all of that work and vision in jeopardy because it's almost unheard of for an assistant producer, my next rung on the ladder, to be part-time. As an assistant producer you are expected, you are required, to be able to film at a moment's notice, and you go home when the filming is done, regardless of what the schedule says, whether it's 6 p.m. or 6 a.m. Everyone in telly accepts this. You stay until the job is done: One Team One Dream. But this is tricky if you have a very angry nanny at home waiting to clock off or a miserable child waiting at nursery to be picked up.

I had also just done my first presenting gig in the form of an authored documentary about women's relation-ships with alcohol for BBC Three. I had loved the process. I had travelled around the country with a brilliant director called Ross, and we had laughed and listened and filmed and danced and drunk with some amazing people. And I had very much hoped to be able to make another one. But, as a colleague had so elegantly told me, pregnancy was career suicide (of course this was completely not true). Which I found so depressing it made me cry on the spot like a child that had dropped an ice cream on to a dog poo.

My income was also very low, which was fine for *me* as I love sandwiches and second-hand clothes and cycling and dying my own hair and stealing my friends' wine, but it was far from enough to support another living, breathing, cloth-wearing person. And with a very low income there was no way that I would be able to afford the childcare that I would need to continue working.

And, to top it all off, my parents were in the middle of a divorce. I felt like one leg of my metaphorical chair had already been kicked away and this new piece of information kicked away another.

So I spun out.

The first person I called was my friend Ele. I think the conversation went something like this: 'Fuck Fuck Fuck Fuck *Fuck*!' This final 'fuck' happened outside Topshop – I remember this because there was a lovely leather jacket in the window and I thought, *Wow, I am window-shopping, how is it possible that I am able to admire a jacket whilst also experiencing such intense stress and drama?* That is commitment to fashion.

For poor Ele, the 'fuck's continued for a full minute before she got bored of my drama. She was, as always, a tower of strength and calm and perspective and support.

Amongst other things, she told me to breathe, to stop pacing and to know that everything was going to be OK. Which gave me enough courage to call my boyfriend.

Now none of my freaking out had anything at all to do with him – I *knew* that I wanted to have children with him, a feeling I'd never had before. But having said that, and although I was excited at feeling such certainty, I was very much imagining rug rats happening in the future, rather than the present right-now-oh-my-God. In the TV industry people generally start thinking about sprogging at around thirty-five years old. So at twenty-eight I felt like a teenager.

I called my boyfriend and suggested that he sit down. He replied that he was fine; he was photocopying.

*OK*, I thought, *here we go*. And I told him, and much to my delight and surprise, he was excited. He was elated. A little bit scared, but mostly overjoyed. Phew. Phew. OK. One worry popped. Fine.

The next twelve hours are a blur but I'm sure there was much calling of parents and drinking of wine (I know, I know) and swearing into oblivion.

The next day I went into work, not sure how the rest of the day, or my life, was going to play out. Because the filming trip I was about to go on was extremely high-adrenalin/adventure and I would need to carry heavy kit, I decided to tell the bosses that I was pregnant. I was offered a place in the development department (the team that comes up with ideas for new shows – fantastically hard, fantastically skilled, and something I was fantastically bad at). It was absolutely the sensible decision and it absolutely sucked. I accepted the offer as, whilst I knew almost nothing about pregnancy and having a baby, I knew that I was probably in for a spot of morning sickness and being halfway up a mountain with a gigantic camera bag strapped to my back probably wasn't the best of ideas. But I did it with the saddest, heaviest of hearts. It felt like the past four years of working my way up the production ladder had been swept away in one tiny moment. Fuck-sticks. Huge, huge fuck-sticks.

So I moved all of my stuff down the corridor to Development. And I will always be hugely grateful to my friend there, Richard Turley (and all the lovely team), for making me laugh every single day. They made it bearable. People can be really sodding great.

Things then progressed quickly, as they do with pregnancy, and I started to feel like I was on a runaway train that I couldn't get off. And because the situation wasn't *quite* overwhelming enough, I had an ectopic scare, which is when the embryo plants itself in your fallopian tube and when it starts to grow it can make the tube explode. It is very dangerous.

I remember the daily visits to the Early Pregnancy Unit to play Hunt the Egg. It was like Easter without the chocolate. No matter how many times they covered my tummy with Ghostbusters goo, the scan just could not detect the foetus. The atmosphere in the waiting room was so thick

174

with anxiety that you could have chopped it up and stewed it. And what a strange experience of polar opposites it was. Half the girls and women in there were desperate for the news that there was no baby inside them, the other half were desperate for the news that there *was* a baby inside them. It all felt so unfair. As I sat there, pretending to read *Take a Break*, I couldn't help but feel abject heartbreak for the girls coming out of the scanning room in floods of tears.

On Christmas Eve my boyfriend and I went for another scan, just after visiting the supermarket to buy a huge fresh festive salmon at Mum's request. As we sat in the hospital for hours and hours waiting to be seen, on an unusually warm December day, we knew that every minute was filling our car with the stench of fish. Which provided us with some welcome comedy relief. Finally they found the embryo hiding behind my coil, and they sent me home. They reassured me that it was better to leave the coil in and that they had seen babies being born holding it in their hand. Strange and cute and creepy all at the same time. So off I went, very glad that my fallopian tube was not going to explode whilst I slept. Very glad indeed.

Over the next few months my belly started to show signs of life but any acceptance of my new fate didn't. And after weeks of moping about, crying on the end of the bed as I woke up and realized again that it wasn't a dream but real, I needed some tough love. A very good and excellent friend gave me a bit of a talking-to. He told me I needed to snap out of it. That I needed to accept things were going to be different to how I had planned. That anyone who held a 'life plan' too tightly was a numpty and that I should expect a few more surprise twists and turns in the future because that was life. That I should accept it, see the beauty in it and choose to be thankful for all that was good and solve all that was bad. He was right. And because he said it with a wonderful balance of toughness and love, it was received loud and clear.

I made myself feel better by doing what I always do when the chips are really down: I went ninja, got organized and ordered more extra hot chips. I bought pregnancy books, I researched everything about early pregnancy and I read about pregnancy nutrition. When life gives you lemons, Google it.

And whilst I was researching pain-free childbirth (I did this almost in jest and then found that it was an *actual* thing) something amazingly brilliant happened. My fairy godfather of a friend, Rob, did something life-changing. Having had me cry on his shoulder at the absurdity of being in my late twenties and yet still not feeling ready to have a child, and having pondered out loud on when the right time to have children really was, considering the social scorn poured on young and old mums alike, he went away and percolated all that we had talked about. Then, because he is a television development demon, he wrote a fantastic pitch for a documentary about that very question – when was the *right* time to become a mum?

Eventually, because he is the kind of person that just makes shit happen, he pitched it to BBC Three and they liked it and commissioned it along with two other programmes – one about dating and one about marriage. So that was a three-part series in the bag, which is a year's worth of work done and dusted. Which, for a freelancer, is pretty flipping wonderfully brilliant. Not only was it secured work for a whole year, but the work allowed me to dive into the lives of other women and the programmes acted as a kind of temperature measure/barometer for what real women of all shapes and sizes and demographics and ages were thinking and feeling today. Which wasn't something I had often seen on television. I will always love BBC Three for commissioning these programmes.

Making a programme about pregnancy had an unexpected benefit – it was extremely cathartic. For three months I travelled the country with a wonderful director called Launa as we searched for mums to talk to about their experience of pregnancy. We met a girl of twelve who was so naive to the reality of what was about to happen that she was without a doubt the most calm and collected mum I met. On the flip side, because she was so heartbreakingly young, her body hadn't finished developing and so the skin on her stomach looked like a tiger had clawed her – but even then, she shrugged it off with little to no concern.

On the other end of the spectrum we filmed with a woman in her forties who had faced huge criticism from others for becoming pregnant via IVF at such a late stage. But like all things, there was so much more to her story. She had wanted to be a mum in her twenties but had suffered many heartbreaking miscarriages. After twelve years of trying to become a mum both naturally and via IVF – remortgaging the house in the process – she and her husband had fallen into a cycle of Just One More Time. They had invested so much emotion and money into becoming parents that each time the IVF wasn't successful they decided they would stop . . . only to both feel that it was worth giving it another go, Just One More Time. And for them, against all odds, it finally worked. And it was twins – wooooop wooooop! And because she kept herself as fit as a fiddle (she had a body like an athlete!), when she did fall pregnant she carried them with as much ease as a girl in her twenties, cherishing every single day that she remained pregnant. In fact, of all the women we filmed with, she was the one who changed my perspective of my own pregnancy 180 degrees. At last I started to feel thankful that I was pregnant and actually a little ashamed at how unappreciative I had been.

I also had one of the most staggeringly amazing filming experiences of my life. I spent some time with an 'alternative' mum who practised yoga every day, and she kindly invited us to be present at the actual birth (a home water one, natch), which we accepted with something close to Utter Glee. And, just as she had planned, it was such a beautifully calm birth that the loudest noise she made resembled that which I make after eating a particularly large burger. I later learned that achieving your desired 'birthing plan' is as rare as spotting a snow leopard in your local supermarket. But her baby's arrival was perfect: a magical, miraculous moment that blew my head off in utter wonder at the unfathomableness of a tiny human coming forth from this lovely woman's belly. And once the baby came out, her mum made everyone tea and toast and jam whilst the new mum held her five-minute-old baby. I remember not really knowing what to say; I think I probably said something awful like 'nice job'. Sheesh.

We also met a brilliantly funny businesswoman called Tjen, who vowed she would be emailing on her BlackBerry during labour and couldn't wait to get back to running her company and would hand her baby over to a nanny the minute she popped out. I later revisited her for a programme investigating breastfeeding and was completely shocked to find that she had, after giving birth, almost immediately handed the company over to her business partner to run (she remained a shareholder and continued to have a hand in the decisions) whilst she stayed at home with her beautiful new baby and worked out when the soonest possible time was that she could get pregnant and have another one. Like everything she did, she dealt with it in a highly efficient and organized way and said outrageous and funny things with a wink of an eye.

And whilst all of this was going on, my body just got on with growing a kid. And the more women I spoke to, the less scared I became. I realized that, until this point, my view of parenthood had been fairly negative. I'd only heard about it in reference to being insane with tiredness, or how painfully expensive children are or how it kills your sex life and spontaneity, or how it's the end of fun holidays and the start of an eternity of purée. It seemed awful. Why would anyone do it, sometimes again and again? How on earth was the world struggling with a population crisis when being a parent was so utterly rubbish? But as I talked to these mums-to-be, they seemed excited at the prospect of being a parent. It was like they knew something I didn't. And that's because they did.

## Things I Learned Whilst Preggers

### You Are Not Eating for Two

I know, I know, isn't that a *HUGE con*?! We grew up being told that, once you get a bun in the oven, you'll be able to establish yourself in Greggs and eat as many buns as you like and you can continue until your only means of exiting is to roll. But this is – deep breath – not fucking true. In fact, all you need is an extra 200–300 calories a day. Which is a piece of toast and a banana. That's it. Yes, you can eat ten doughnuts on the trot and, yes, you can start the day with a hot sausage-roll sandwich, *but* any extra weight you put on, you will have to lose after you've given birth – or not, depending on exactly how many fucks you give, which could be zero. There is no magical post-pregnancy fairy that does it for you. And anyone encouraging you to 'Just chill and let go' or who says, 'Oh sod it, just enjoy yourself and have another Krispy Kreme,' does not have to go to for a run with you at 5.30 a.m. before the baby wakes up or pay for the childcare whilst you go to the gym or be there when you can't put on any of your old trousers or wipe the tears when you are trying to deal with the identity shift of being a mother whilst also not feeling good about yourself.

I learned the hard way that, no, I was *not* eating for two in *amount*, but in *responsibility*. I realized that being preggers is the time to laugh in the face of Five a Day and go for As Many as Possible a Day because you are growing another human. And that, because the uterus expands and pushes upwards, your stomach's capacity becomes much smaller, so little and often works best. (Wow, I have had some painful experiences of ignoring this and just powering through with burger and chips and pudding and cheese. Not to be recommended, especially if you are in a public place that doesn't appreciate a pregnant women curled up in the foetal position moaning into her napkin or being a little bit sick.)

**Morning Sickness**

Firstly, this doesn't happen only in the morning – it can be any time of the day. Yup, suck on that. Also, ignore all the righteous food crap I just wrote. When it came to morning sickness there was only one thing that worked for me:

pepperoni pizza. A whole pizza. And if anyone else wanted a slice, they'd have to think carefully about whether they wanted the use of their arm afterwards. For my first pregnancy I was such a smug twat about morning-sickness cures – for some reason chopped-up melon worked a treat for me – but the chickens came home to roost for my second child. I tried chopped melon but it took me from nausea to hovering over the loo sweating like a butcher at Christmas. And then it hit me like a slap: pizza. And I was in Sainsbury's and home and eating it quicker than you could say 'melon shmelon'. I almost didn't even cook it.

## Pregnancy Hangover

Morning sickness gets a lot of airtime but the pregnancy hangover was a new discovery for me. I was lucky in that my experience of morning sickness was OK – I was never actually physically sick. But the hangover? Wow. I think it was my body's way of telling me to Chill the Fuck Out and sit down. It came in waves so thick and fast that I would be walking along the road and know that if I didn't find somewhere to be horizontal within four minutes I would have to lie on the pavement and risk being arrested. It's annoying because you can justify taking time off work for morning sickness but, for my first pregnancy anyway, I didn't feel I could stay at home for being 'tired'. It felt so pathetic. So I would take naps in the disabled toilet or pretend to be writing detailed notes when I was in fact having a very tiny sleep at my desk.

For baby number two, I realized that this was ridiculous and watched a lot of daytime television and hit the deck the minute I felt the urge to sleep, like a cat in a sunbeam. This was of course made easier by being a freelancer as I only had myself to answer to and I often said 'Hell yes, take this morning off'. What a nice modern boss.

## Don't Lift Anything Heavy

Feeling sure of my Bruce Lee-like strength, I completely ignored the advice to avoid lifting anything heavy. Which was very, very silly. Because I gave myself piles. I have always joked about piles. They are in my comedy chat. And because the universe had heard my tasteless jokes, it decided to give me a little gift. So after helping my mum move house, and carrying a small(ish) cupboard plus about five suitcases down three flights of stairs, the nerves in my bottom decided to protest. I was eight months pregnant and with the weight of an almost-ready-to-drop baby and the unexpected load of furniture, my body gave me a lesson in ignoring good advice.

## Say No to Maxi Dresses

I'm not sure who started it but the maxi-dress trend for pregnant women is perplexing. Why, when you are already a challenging shape for clothes, would you wear something that, at the best of times, is almost impossible to pull off? I attempted a maxi dress at about seven months pregnant but knew instantly that I looked like a Dalek lost in haberdashery. Because of the protruding bump, the maxi dress creates a tent, so I looked like I was ready to provide shelter for a small family on a rainy day. Maxi dresses are the worst thing to happen to pregnant women since pregnant women were told they could eat for two. The bump is beautiful. Don't hide it.

### Train for Childbirth

This may sound nuts – particularly considering how often I was poleaxed by the aforementioned pregnancy hangovers – but I didn't understand why I was being told to put my feet up and see the nine months of pregnancy as a time to chill out. What? I am about to *give birth* – that is one of the most physically challenging, exhausting activities a woman will ever do, and it might result in some kind of surgical procedure, and therefore shouldn't I be as fit as I can to make the recovery faster? Also, surely the bump is going to get big and heavy and so I am going to need a strong back to carry that load? And surely, if my body is about to take a beating from any of the many wonderful side effects of pregnancy, then I need it to be in the best possible condition to cope with those? So, once I had overcome the battering of the first three months, I carried on exercising, although definitely dialling it down, and found out that the new advice to pregnant women is to carry on with anything they've already been doing but to adjust it as the bump gets bigger (unless it is something extreme like marathon running or shark wrestling or anything of that nature). (And I learned that it's not a good idea to do mini-trampoline classes as you wet yourself. Yeah, I did this and, yeah, I wet myself. Yeah.)

So I carried on going to the gym, trying to ignore the looks of confusion as I waddled around with a gigantic bump (at that stage I was mostly walking on an incline on the treadmill and doing very light weights). I am aware this sounds hideously smug – but I suppose when I was pregnant I felt annoyed for myself and other pregnant women that the advice they are given (i.e. chill out, babes, you're preggers) is lovely to hear but doesn't serve us in the end when we're left, literally, holding the baby.

## Childbirth

Finally, the bun had finished cooking and, whilst some people seemed to think it was nerve-wracking that the birth was going to be filmed, I was more nervous about pushing the equivalent of a lemon out of my nostril in the presence of half a dozen perfect strangers, some of which who would sporadically put their hands up my lady tunnel. By now my stomach protruded so much that it entered the room before me. Even at the end stages, when I'd had all my scans and *seen* the child within, I found pregnancy a very, very surreal experience. Some women connect very intensely to their bump and revel that it contains their unborn child – but I didn't find that. I just watched it with perplexed fascination. Having never fantasized about having children I found that

I wasn't sentimental about the bump. For me, the fun was in the abstract notion that it was growing without any input from me. Yes, I was eating broccoli and trying to exercise, but other than that I wasn't helping at all. The miracle of life was occurring as I sat and watched the telly or stared out of the window on the bus. And even when a tiny elbow or foot would kick me it remained so surreal that my head struggled to accept it was a real human.

Thanks to hypnobirthing, I was feeling more calm about the birth, having previously been scared of nothing more – thanks in part to someone who told me that it was similar to the end of *Braveheart* when he is hung, drawn and quartered, or someone else who told me it's like trying to pull a melon out of your nose. For anyone scared of giving birth I highly recommend hypnobirthing, which aims to reconnect the mother with the natural process of childbirth, rather than the medicalized screaming-in-pain nightmare that we are led to expect. Because we are braced for a hideous experience, all of our muscles are tense and it makes getting a baby out even more of a challenge.

For some good reasons, which I won't attempt to fully explain here, hypnobirthing teaches that it is possible to have a calm birth. It absolutely does not guarantee this but it does give you the tools to have the most peaceful birth possible. The best bit is the wonderfully calming meditation CDs. I used to listen to them in the bath, trying to get into a lovely floppy, relaxed state whilst also imaging my cervix 'opening like a flower' (tee-hee).

By the time the bump was at max capacity I felt ready to Do This Shit. I was in a calm(er) place about getting the human out of my vagina and also about the prospect of being a parent. So my due date arrived and we paused filming.

And I waited, and waited. And waited some more.

After ten days of watching and waiting and measuring and scanning, we all got bored and the doctors started to worry that there wasn't enough amniotic fluid being produced. So they decided to induce me, which involved admitting me into hospital and putting a pipette of synthetic pig sperm inside me. Not kidding. Well, this could be an urban myth but, even in my labour-induced haze, I'm pretty sure this is what they told me. And so, in preparation for this slightly science-fiction solution working its magic, I sent my boyfriend off to Greggs to buy six doughnuts. Because I felt that, if I was about to run my metaphorical marathon, then I was going to have to give myself one hell of a carrot.

One of the methods I had used to ease the fear of childbirth was to promise myself unadulterated baked-good gluttony. And I know it sounds pretty unorthodox but it worked a treat. Many people told me that, whilst interesting in theory, there was no way I would be able to stomach a doughnut during labour. And they were so very, very wrong. My boyfriend bought me six different varieties and I ate all six. And when I dropped one on to the floor, I picked it up (still wired to the monitor) and ate it. That is doughnut love. (I did this again with my second child and found that it actually made me look forward to his birth. I ignored the fact that I had planned a caesarean so wasn't technically doing the labour marathon. But a deal is a deal. Birth = doughnuts.)

The iced buns flowed but the bun in the oven did not. She just would not come out. It was obviously very cosy in there. So I was given a stretch and sweep. I sodding hated this. Hated it. Essentially, the midwife tries to manually open your cervix to start things off. To add to the hideousness, because my cervix is extremely high and tilted back, I essentially had to be fisted in order for it to be accessed. Mmm-hmm.

As you can imagine, I have enjoyed other activities more. But what I did learn through that experience is that YOU are in control. This kind of procedure hurts significantly less if you are relaxed. And that means you have to tell the midwife when to move her hand. This definitely takes more time but if the midwife is a good 'un she won't be cross if you are assertive about how you'd like this done. It's *your* vagina. I wish I had been more vocal about this.

This sadly didn't work so they let me sit back on my bouncy Pilates ball and stare out of the window, listening to relaxing music and putting into practice everything I'd learned in hypnobirthing. Very gradually the contractions started to get stronger, but by staying relaxed I felt as though it was manageable.

Until it wasn't.

I then *demanded* some gas and air. It made me a bit bonkers. For a start, it made my voice incredibly low. I remember thinking to myself that the last thing I needed at this moment in my life was to sound like Barry White.

And then I Lost It.

I started laughing manically because the pain was so bad, which made my boyfriend take away my gas, because he thought it was making me hysterical. So I would try to get it back. And when I say get it back, I mean grab it back with an expression similar to the scary children in *The Shining*.

I then became extremely disorientated and wasn't sure of where I was or who the other people were and demanded that everyone except my boyfriend leave the room whilst I sorted my shit out. He was then left alone with a hysterically laughing and crying loon bouncing on a ball and clawing at him like a rabid cat.

So, after I had calmed down and got into a manageable flow, the midwives decided it was time to check me (yeah, another pleasant situation where the midwife exclaims 'Gosh, you DO have a JOLLY HIGH cervix, don't you?!'. I was never sure how to respond to this) and then delivered the news that I had dilated one centimetre. One tiny, weedy, sodding centimetre.

I was a broken woman. It felt like getting to the end of a marathon to be told you had, in fact, only completed the first five per cent of the race. I could not believe it.

And then something really fun happened. They manually broke my waters. Naively I assumed that there must be some kind of cool technology or drug for doing this. Yeahhh, not so much. It is prehistoric. I don't want to scare anyone but they also say that the truth will set you free, and gosh I wish I had known beforehand. Then at least I could have engaged the 'slow and steady and only with my exhale and only when I'm ready' technique. That would have actually been OK.

So, you ready? They basically used a knitting needle. And because I was not expecting this and was high as a flipping kite and because the entrance to my cervix is harder to find than the meaning of life it was a bit of a fight. And, like the checks and the stretch 'n' sweeps, I wish I had been more assertive (tricky when you are almost tripping) and asked for the needle to only be moved when I was breathing deeply. And so my waters broke, which resulted in a very unsatisfying '*shpler*' of liquid. I had hoped for a brilliantly dramatic SHPLOOOSSSHHH, like in the films, but of course that only happens in films.

So once again, we waited. And I got back on the gas 'n' air. Still my cervix refused to play ball. Then, because time was now of the essence, they brought out the big guns. The glorious anaesthetist administered the glorious epidural, because the drugs I was about to be given would take my contractions into the stratosphere, and I praised the Lord for modern medicine and pronounced several times that I loved her, which, she later told me, happens to her a lot. It was magical.

After a while, it was time for another check and, you've guessed it, there'd been no progress at all. So the doctor very delicately – and slightly nervously, as my birth plan had originally been to have a home water birth – suggested a Caesarean. Before he had even finished his sentence I chimed in with, 'Yes, yes, do it, do it.' Because I was out of doughnuts, my throat hurt from all the laughing/crying and I was really very tired. Much to my surprise, the fear and risk of having a major operation was the last thing on my mind – all I could think about was, after being awake for nearly thirty-five hours, I might get a chance to have a little shut-eye whilst they were prepping. Priorities.

The next bit is a blur but somehow I ended up in one of those blue backless surgery gowns that shows your bum in the operating room, with my boyfriend sitting by my head and the director balancing precariously on a stool behind me, trying to find the best angle to capture enough to tell the story but not so much that it would put people off their dinner. And, because the atmosphere was so calm and everyone seemed to know what they were doing, I started to drift off into a delicious snooze. My poor boyfriend was given the job of trying to keep me awake but it was an uphill battle. I was so stoned with tiredness and the doctors were so skilled and gentle that I didn't even really feel them rummaging about. It was very serene.

And then she emerged. A tiny, bloody, mucusy, crying human. The nurses gave her a little rub-down and then placed her on to my chest. Then they told me the little human was a girl.

Much like the start of this whole process, I felt that my being was falling from my body at 100 mph. The incredible mind-blowing information that I now had a daughter and seeing her beautiful, beautiful tiny face, and feeling a wave of emotion that words will never be able to truly describe and because I am extremely overdramatic at the best of times I thought that I might explode into a thousand pieces through the sheer intensity of the experience. So I started hyperventilating (I have never hyperventilated before or since) and had to hand her over to my boyfriend whilst I chilled the fuck out. He held her. He kissed her face. And I cried and cried.

And because of my lack of connection with the bump and my acute fear of being a parent, I had slightly expected to suffer from either postnatal depression or struggle to bond with the baby. I was so thankful that this didn't happen. It was pretty much instant raging, passionate love at first sight.

So what did I learn from this experience? Well, for anyone reading this who happens to be about to sprog, here's my advice:

- Research your birth options. Write a birth plan. Talk it through with your midwife. Give it your best shot. But be prepared to chuck it out of the window the minute your circumstances change. Or if you just feel that maybe you don't quite fancy 'breathing' the baby out now it feels like someone is wringing out your innermost parts with a giant fist, and you'd actually quite like some heavy-duty drugs and to be woken up when it's all over, thank you very much. There's no shame in this. Equally, if it's really important for you to have a natural birth even when you're being pressured to go for the 'easy' option and sign up for painkillers, stick to your guns. It's your body. You get to choose.

- Never feel bad if you don't achieve your 'ideal' birth. Very few people do. It is a messy, sometimes brutal, business and it is unpredictable. But ultimately it's one day out of your life. Whereas your journey as a parent is beginning right now and will carry on every day for the rest of your entire life.

- Think very carefully about who you want in the birth room with you. For some people it will be their partner; others may feel they'd be the least relaxing person imaginable to have about the place. Again it's your choice: you might ask a friend, your mother or a trusted relative. In my case it was a film crew, which was possibly a little unorthodox.

- Remember, doughnuts are your friends.

# 7. Letter to My Face: Teeth, Brows, Skin, Make-Up, Ageing, Self-Improvement, A Day a Week

*Dearest Face,*

*Eating, smiling, crying, kissing, vomiting, biting, snoring, snorting, smelling. You really are a busy bee. I work you to the bone. If I am lucky enough to reach a ripe old age, I will probably look like that old tangerine at the bottom of the fruit bowl. But whilst there is definitely a part of me that bows to society's adoration of youth there is also a part of me, a part that I am trying to nurture, that embraces and adores signs of a life lived with passion and expression and laughing and guffawing and licking and loving. It's a shame that as men grow older society says they grow wiser and more distinguished, whereas women seem to become obsolete and haggard. (That is, of course, utter bollocks. As women grow older they become equally distinguished and wise – and caring and warm and clever and beautiful.)*

*So bosh on, lovely face! Go forth! They say that eyes are the windows to the soul – well, fling them wide open and let people in! Life is too short not to smile until your cheeks ache and frown like you're trying to crack a nut with your temples and laugh until your contact lenses fall out and contort until you are blue in the face.*

# Teeth

Teeth are weird. They are, essentially, our highest-maintenance body part. They need flossing and mouthwashing and brushing morning and night. They sometimes need braces and bridge work and whitening and filling and dentures and hygienists and procedures so painful that I don't want to write them down. Frankly they let us down. I recently found out what veneers were and how they are done. It's like something out of a horror film. The dentist files the teeth into a spike, which must be brain-meltingly painful. He then slots razor-sharp enamel covers on to those filed teeth to give a perfect white smile. But because these enamel covers are pushed up into your gums, it feels like a dozen little knives are poking you all day long until it settles. I mean, oh my God. Is this real? Yes. It is. And it's really popular. When I was in America several of my colleagues had gone through this procedure and were mainlining children's teething gel (in America this is so strong that it numbs your entire face within two seconds – which is probably why it isn't allowed in the UK) so that they wouldn't weep during meetings. Wow. The lengths we go to for a set of white teeth.

And whilst I know that it's hugely important, I find brushing my teeth fantastically boring and so does my daughter. Every morning I have to ask her three, four, twelve times to brush her teeth – because it is more boring than almost any other activity. Even doing a wee has a bigger pay-off. I now watch TED Talks whilst I do it so that I don't feel like it's a huge waste of my short and precious time on earth. I also shop on Etsy. Which is perhaps less nurturing but I do have some great rainbow cushions as a consequence.

In essence, teeth are a pain but if you want to avoid tooth pain then you have to submit to their will. I am amazed that in 2016 'they' haven't found a more time-efficient way to keep them healthy. From the cradle to the grave, teeth are a pain in the arse.

Other than sneaking into my mother's bedroom to play in her make-up drawer (a no-go zone) and doing a Pat-from-*Eastenders* with the blue eyeshadow that came free with my *Just Seventeen*, my first experience of facial augmentation was braces. Great big bloody silver train-tracks, top and bottom, each with little hooks connected by multicoloured elastic bands, because clearly my braces weren't prominent enough without them.

Like all rites of passage, the idea of them was quite exciting, like getting glasses or your first training bra. Some of the older girls in the school had braces and when I was fifteen and had my orthodontist appointment set in the diary it meant I was also one of the older girls. Wicked.

I think this is a perfect example of 'Be careful what you wish for.' I hope and pray that nowadays the method for putting on braces is more advanced because it felt like something from the days when people brushed their teeth with sticks and thought that couples therapy was beating your wife with a club using only one hand instead of two.

So on they went. They were a sight to behold. Even though I knew I looked pretty terrifying, the main focus was trying to manage the intense ache as my teeth were very, very slowly being pulled in different directions. Even remembering it now gives me face-ache.

The intensity of the pain would calm after a few days and an inordinate amount of painkillers, but then it would start again when they were tightened a few months later. And this magical cycle went on for *three years*. (But at least they gave me different coloured elastic bands. Double thumbs.) I have to admit the length of time was entirely down to me. One year, about fifteen months after having them installed, I was on holiday with my family, and my brother and I were sitting on some grass waiting for my parents to finish chatting to other parents. (Don't you hate it when they tell you 'It's time to go' and then stand in the frickin' doorway talking for thirty minutes? Yeah, I do that to my kids now.)

Well. We were bored and surrounded by long grass and so obviously I felt it was necessary to pick the long grass and thread the blades through each of the gaps in my braces, thus joining my upper and lower jaws in a rustic Hannibal Lecter effect. Which made my brother laugh. And so I then pulled them so that my lips would move in a weird way. Which made my brother laugh. And then I tried to see exactly how much grass I could fit into my braces because I thought that would also make my brother laugh. Which it did, but it also pulled the wire out from the brackets, so I was left with a mouthful of razor-sharp, entirely ineffectual metal boxes on each of my teeth. Bloody brilliant. So, because my teeth were relatively new to their amended position, an entire year's worth of eye-, nose-, cheek- and brain-ache was undone in a matter of days as my teeth – which had clearly been very happy in their original state – went back to where they started. Thank you very much.

When I returned to the orthodontist he informed me that we would have to start again. Nearly from scratch. From lots of pain to no gain back to lots of pain. And that is why I had braces for three whole formative years. Even to this day I will always feel affection for my boyfriends of that time for seeing beyond my mouth of metal and yellow elastic bands.

But now, because of this ridiculous saga, I truly appreciate and value my teeth. And even though she rolls her eyes and tells me to put the kettle back on, I tell this to my daughter. And because dental work is time-consuming, expensive and painful, I have now invested in an electric toothbrush so powerful it could get chewing gum off the pavement. Pretty much anything to avoid veneers is a bonus I think.

## Brows

No self-respecting teenager of the nineties has a fully functioning browline that doesn't need daily colouring in with an eyebrow pencil. A bit like the message that women must all look like depressed crack addicts to be sexy, or the noughties trend for a full Brazilian, in the nineties we were told that eyebrows just weren't an option for a woman who wanted to interact with civilized society. So my next experience of face augmentation was a regular violent assault on my eyebrows.

Naturally my mother, in a chorus of other mothers around the country, chimed that it wasn't a good idea to remove every eyebrow hair except three but, like all teens we ignored their wisdom because everyone knows that older women don't know anything and are witches anyway. So we all plucked like our lives depended on it and hoped that we would end up looking like depressed crack addicts but instead ended up with two anorexic slugs crawling listfully across our faces. For ever.

Of course now we have the Brow Goddess Cara Delevingne to teach us the error of our plucking ways. Which is great but too late, because as every female contemporary of mine knows, if you over-pluck your eyebrows they don't sodding grow back. So thanks, fashion editors, yet another must-have feature that we simply *can't* have.

I would like to thank modern make-up for throwing me a life ring. Having realized I could actually draw my brows back on, I bought a pencil and started colouring. I did this, without consulting another human, like a toddler trying to draw a set of caterpillars, for months.

Then one day I was pottering around in a department store and was approached by a particularly assertive and particularly confused-looking make-up salesperson. I think her first question was 'Why are your eyebrows ginger when your hair is blonde and your eyelashes are brown?' I felt like showing her my pubic hair to see if that held the answer. She then gave me an angled brow brush and a pot of light brown eyeshadow that was the right colour and texture. She explained that powder is much less harsh than a pencil and would not be so obvious. She showed me how to apply in an upward motion and how to create a natural but flattering arch and how to brush it out a little afterwards to create a more subtle effect. It's amazing how, sometimes, it's the little details that make a big difference. Yes, I might be follicularly challenged but with the power of an assertive observer and some education I kissed goodbye to my two little orange friends and walked into the sunset with eyebrows worthy of a high five.

## Skin

Here are a few things I've learned about loving the skin we're in:

### Spots

One of the things I didn't realize aged sixteen was that spots don't stop after you're a teenager. Well, they didn't for me. Woop, flipping woop. But I am my own worst enemy in this area as I hack, hack, hack at them like a rabid archaeologist and I turn something that was tiny and minding its own business into a monster of angry pain and wrath. I just can't help myself. And, like so many things in life, my head will be telling me 'This isn't a good idea, you should not do this,' and yet the impulse is so strong that I do it anyway. Kids, take it from someone who knows: this is a Bad Idea. Leave those spots alone.

## Skin Myths

Some 'golden rules' of skincare are invented by skincare companies to make you buy more stuff. They say one of the golden rules is to never go to sleep with make-up on, but I think that's rubbish. I have spent the best part of two decades religiously adhering to this rule but recently, with two kids and both a love of going out late and a need to get up early to do the school run, I have, very occasionally, been going to bed without taking it all off. And, well, mostly, the world keeps turning and, after a good wash in the morning, normal service resumes. Having broken the spell of this myth I have been experimenting over the past year and I would say that, if I haven't got much make-up on, I can get away with this about once or twice a week before my skin starts to show the effect of the lack of love. Of course every skin is different but I think that my skin likes a break from being scrubbed and slathered in products. So to all of those women frantically wet-wiping, cotton-woolling, washing, exfoliating and moisturizing their faces every single night, I say to you: give yourself two nights off, and maybe more depending on how tetchy your face is. It's bliss. It's like being a man.

# Water

In interviews with models and celebs and women with disposable income and a 'capsule wardrobe' (I still don't really know what this is and why anyone would want to keep clothes in a capsule) there is often some conversation about how they keep their skin looking so beauteous and the reply is often something annoying, like 'I drink tons and tons of water, eat organic and sleep at least eight hours every day' when in fact it's almost certainly thanks to monthly £200 Harley Street facials, acid peels and any number of strange treatments (the most horrifying new one currently is a procedure that injects the patient's face with their own blood – yes, this is real). Anyway, even though the standard *'water, sleep and kale'* answer is often a porky-pie, my mother *has* always told me that drinking lots of water is good and I am starting to think it might be a good idea to begin listening to her wonderful wisdom. And since I've upped my water intake I have noticed some fabulous changes:

1. I pee more often, which is always fun and means I have more time to reply to emails and texts.
2. I have a bit more energy.
3. My skin sometimes looks a bit nicer.
4. I have turned into one of those vexing people who waxes lyrical about how fabulous my new BPA-free silicone-coated glass water bottle is.
5. My friends invite me out less.

I have been flying a lot recently for work and used to wonder why other people were necking gallons of water on the flight whilst I was ordering my fifth G & T and tucking into another packet of extra-high-salt crisps. After suffering the consequences of this salt and booze assault (walking around New York feeling like I had life-threatening flu) I realized that perhaps my in-flight entertainment needed some adjusting. So now I drink water in between my G & Ts (baby steps) and eat cheese (baby steps).

## Make-Up

I hope that my daughter loves herself enough to walk around as happy as a hamster without a scrap of make-up on, *but* should she be in the mood for some face decoration I would love to have taught her a few basics (which she will then cross-reference with an online tutorial and realize that I know absolutely nothing about make-up).

YouTube tutorials are the best thing to happen to personal adornment since we realized that foundation should be the same colour as our skin and probably not stop exactly at the jawline without being blended (yeah, I rocked this look for years). Ninety per cent of the time the tutorials are fun and helpful and add to the joy of being a woman. They have taught me how to do a sixties liner flick, how to backcomb my hair and how to do a smokey eye whilst avoid looking like Aunt Margaret after a long night out on the razz.

But sometimes the YouTube tutorials are depressing. There are too many to mention that reinforce the idea that a girl needs to be made-up to go about her everyday business. I have found some that teach girls how to achieve an 'everyday' look for pottering about the shops that takes *forty minutes*. Forty actual life minutes. That you can never get back. Do you know how much fun or sleep or masturbation you could have in that time?! LOTS. Surely, if you're popping out to buy some bananas, you either exit au naturel or shmoosh some foundation over your red bits, swish some bronzer over your protruding bits and swizzle your eyebrows into place and then you're good to go? That is achievable in *five* golden minutes. Done and done.

It pains me to think that young girls really would spend forty of their precious earth minutes every day preparing themselves just to leave the house to buy some garlic bread. But I was reminded by a teenager recently that we now live in the age of the selfie, and so she felt she needed to be prepared at any moment. Yes, she was just going to the local playground to loaf about *but* there was a good chance someone would take a photograph and that point in time would be immortalized for ever and seen by every human being she had ever met and quite a few she hadn't. I think I underestimated how much pressure young girls are under to look fabulous at *every possible moment*, which probably explains why there are an unfathomable amount of make-up tutorials on YouTube.

As with all things that befuddle the older generation, I am sure that there will be a beautiful silver lining to this depressing thought, and I hope that it looks something like a full circle, where girls choose to embrace their natural selves, if only to give themselves an extra thirty minutes in their cosy, warm beds.

I think one of the most useful and healthiest phrases I want my daughter to have at her fingertips is *'Does it really matter?'* If she wakes up with a crap spot, if her hair is having a crap day, if it's a laundry day and the only thing left to wear is her crap onesie, I hope her automatic thought is: *'Does it really matter?'*

Because no, it doesn't. It might be annoying but it's totally fine. There are some things that *really* matter: handing schoolwork in on time, handing career work in on time, turning up to school/work/dates on time. Paying your parking fine on time. Paying your tax bill on time. Smiling at people who are having a shit day. Inviting those people round for a cup of tea and listening to them. Replying to emails from people who are having a rubbish day. Being honest with people who have spinach in their teeth. Remembering your friend has a big exam, big date or court hearing. Sending a thoughtful text or calling someone you think might be lonely. Keeping your heart healthy. Trying new things. Calling your mum. Eating carrots. Those matter.

I wish I had known this when I was growing up. It is the emotional equivalent of popping a boil. It feels amazing when I don't like my skin/clothes/weight/mood to be able to ask myself *Does it really matter?* If the answer's no, then chin up, bosh on and have a glorious day. (I achieve this at least four out of ten times I try it – but I'm confident that will increase as I get older and wiser.)

## Ageing

Speaking of being wise, let's talk about witches. Back to fairy tales again. Why are all the evil characters old women? Yeah, I know, blew me away too when someone pointed that out to me. The old witch in the tower holding the young and beautiful and stupid (but who cares, because she's a hottie) Rapunzel hostage. The old jealous stepmother of Cinderella, the young and stupid (but, most importantly, beautiful) girl in need of pity and saving. And who could forget the wrinkled old hag that tricked poor, innocent, idiotic (but, most importantly, beautiful) Sleeping Beauty into being pricked by a needle? (And then there's Hansel and Gretel, proving that old women are manipulative child-killers.)

In short, young people are silly sausages but beautiful and innocent; men are heroes and always have a solution for any problem even if it's as simple as having a snog; old men are wise and kind and regal and powerful; old women are toothless warty old hags that lie and cheat and manipulate. Is it any wonder that we fight against signs of ageing as though our self-worth depended on it?

I wonder how many women grow into old age and feel surprised that they are more thoughtful, wise and kind; that it's easier to make good decisions; that they still feel interesting and interested and switched on and relevant; that they have not sprouted a warty nose; and that they have a Freedom Pass and prefer that to a broom (huge wedgie issues). I know that my own mother, who is about to turn seventy, finds all this a pleasant surprise.

## Self-Improvement

So. Being a woman is very fun. We get to play with how we look and, as long as it stays in the joy arena and avoids the anxiety arena, it's brilliant. But with all of these things how do we ensure that we are engaging happily and not because we don't feel valuable enough without it? Make-up, jewellery, Botox, tucks, lifts, fillers, slicing 'n' dicing . . . where is the line?

Well, I believe that we set our own lines. For some people, a slick of eyeliner is over the line and for others a surgeon drawing lines on their body pre-op isn't over the line. I think it's about why and who for and how much. With the boundaries changing all the time, how can we really place a judgement on what is OK and what isn't? Even five years ago Botox was frowned upon. Now it's a socially accepted way to deal with your lines and talked about openly by women who were previously slating others. Even something as dramatic as surgery, once hidden and lied about, is becoming accepted.

I used to say that the boundary is when you've gone beyond highlighting what you have and start adding what you don't. But I don't any more and here is why:

- I don't think it's our job as feminists to set the boundaries for each other.
- I don't think it's helpful to judge women who step outside *our* line.
- Harshly judging how other women look is often rooted in our own insecurity, fear of something we're not familiar with or just good ol' smuggery. Let's not do it to each other – it's shit.
- Making snippy comments about someone's bad plastic surgery or botched lip fillers might be fun for five seconds but then you are the person who makes mean bitchy comments about someone's bad plastic surgery or botched lip fillers. And you have to live with you pretty much all the time.
- The person who has had the bad surgery almost certainly knows they don't look quite right and probably already feels pretty awful and if they don't then hurray, I hope they never do, because what the world doesn't need is one more woman feeling bad about herself because of the way she looks.

If anything we should be naming and shaming the plastic surgeons who slice and dice their clients well beyond anything reasonable. Why aren't they abiding by their Hippocratic oath and refusing to operate on someone who is clearly going to look like they've been in a wind tunnel for too long? They're the ones we should be talking about on Twitter. But they pocket their tens of thousands of pounds and disappear into the background whilst their victims/clients have to carry the greed on their faces for the rest of their lives.

Last year I did a project in LA and was struck by how many women have *very* obvious plastic surgery, sometimes so much that it's hard to look at. The message it sends isn't one of comfort and security and beauty and joy, it's the exact opposite. So – here I go judging – what I don't understand is why *so many* have done this? I don't get it. You can tell that they were gorgeous women before, so why mess with that? Is the fear of being old so bad that it's worth the risk? Clearly, yes. Which makes me sad. How have we got ourselves into such a state that beautiful women will mutilate themselves just to avoid being thought of as a bit older? Holy cow, it's hard to fathom. For anyone thinking that feminism is outdated and defunct, go to LA and have a look at all the women who would rather have their bodies mauled than lose their aesthetic value.

And why do women have this fear of losing their aesthetic value in the first place? Why does society place such incredibly high value on our looks? It's clear that a huge factor in this is how, historically, our physical appeal has been vital to our survival. Broadly speaking, men have chosen their mate based on their attractiveness and women have chosen their mate based on how well they can provide. So, without the same education and opportunities to earn money as men, a woman's desire to look good wasn't so much as vanity as a way to ensure her security. But now we can be surgeons, judges, teachers, business leaders, chefs, athletes, candlestick makers; we can vote, have our own mortgage, drive, run marathons or even just assemble a packed lunch for our kids whilst fielding a conference call from work and hunting for a lost PE kit at the same time. We can do *anything*. So what on earth are we doing worrying about whether we have a retroussé nose or a glassy-smooth forehead? Who are we doing this *for*?

Which brings me back to the pressure of the internet. If we thought women were under pressure before, it's now been unquantifiably magnified by the internet, which is essentially a gigantic whirling mirror to human nature that we have unleashed and are trying to work out how to tame. When I was growing up, I only needed to worry about look-ing presentable at very specific times: occasional parties (when someone might have a disposable camera and the resulting pictures often remained unseen by everyone other than a handful of people) and maybe Christmas Day, when Mum would make me put on a dress and brush my hair. Whereas for girls now, the pressure that someone will whip out their phone and immortalize their appearance is almost 24/7. The pictures are posted on Facebook or Instagram for all the world to see again, and again and again.

So I think it's even more vital that we instil in our girls a sense of worth beyond how they look. I want my daughter to grow up with *more* self-esteem and *more* brain-time to think about *more* wondrous things and to have *more* freedom to shove on a T-shirt and jeans if she feels like it.

Because she's worth it.

## A Day a Week

I once worked out that I spent nearly *a day a week* (what the fuckity fuck!) making myself look fairly average: waxing, shaving, plucking, washing and colouring and styling my hair, buying and styling outfits, clipping nails, filing nails, painting nails, taking paint off nails, cleansing and toning (and the occasional face mask), buffing, exfoliating, putting make-up on and wiping it off, smearing on serum, slathering on moisturizer . . . All of this takes up rather a lot of time. A day a week adds up to fifty-two days a year. Time is the most valuable thing we have and so I'd say that was rather expensive. And, whilst adding up the time I spent each week was quite depressing, it was even worse when I looked at the list of other possible lady-admin activities. Here is but a glimpse of the giant beauty-industry iceberg: tanning, extensions, threading, Botox, mani/pedi, blow-drying, vajazzles, lipo, bleaching, etc.

And not only is this a black hole for our hard-earned cash but, worse, it is a huge chunk of lady-brain-time. Imagine being a boy and just being able to brush your teeth, run your hands through your hair, put on a T-shirt and jeans or suit and walk out of the door. And never giving your physical appearance another thought throughout the day. Wowzers.

I do absolutely love getting dressed up. I adore clothes and I am a gigantic fan of a massage/facial/blow-dry/being touched in any way at all. But I do think that the *amount* of time it takes for the average woman, on a daily basis, to feel confident enough to leave the house is fairly bonkers. And while many of us enjoy some aspects of lady-admin some of the time, how many of us do it because we think, sometimes rightly, that we *have* to do it. Think of all the collective lady-time and lady-brain-space and lady-finances that are given to the tanning industry alone. Especially considering that most women look significantly more beautiful sporting their natural skin tone than they do with orange streaks on their wrists and ankles.

I did this tanning dance for *years,* hoping in vain that no one would notice my brown palms (like a Care Bear) and orange feet (like I have a thyroid problem) until I realized that I always, always noticed it on others. My finest moment was when I was twenty-three and my friend invited me on a holiday of a lifetime. Her Austrian boyfriend had invited a gaggle of fun people to his home (which was like the headquarters of a James Bond baddie – at the push of a button one of the walls would sink into the floor to reveal a beautiful mountain view) for a New Year's party. I was so single and so ready to mingle. And so that I would wow the boys into a frenzied state of desire I decided to have my first spray tan. What a fantastic time to experiment with spray tans. And yes, you've guessed it, it was a disaster. I left the salon looking like I'd just come back from a holiday in the Maldives, and twenty-four hours later I arrived in Salzburg looking like I was wearing a Gruffalo onesie. And I spent four days laughing it off, making it seem as though I was totally comfortable with how silly it looked, whereas the truth was I was mortified.

And so, about three years later and after many similar experiences, I finally threw in the tanning towel and accepted that it was OK not to look like I'd just flown in from St Tropez because I had never flown in from St Tropez and neither had anyone I was hanging out with. I was a runner working in the dark windowless basement of the old BBC building in Shepherd's Bush and it was OK not to have a golden tan. And it was one of the best things I've ever done. It immediately freed up *so much time and money* that I now feel highly vexed at *all the time and money* I spent standing spreadeagled in my bathroom waiting to dry, smelling like a biscuit and feeling like a total arse. Since writing this I have actually returned to the dark side as I've discovered a tanning spray that is lightening quick and doesn't make me smell like biscuits. I smell like crisps instead.

# 8. Letter to My Ears: Music, Listening, Silence, Unhelpful Things to Hear, Talking Dirty

*Listen up, Ears,*

*You've been pretty easy-going, so thank you. You keep the hair out of my face and you've given me Michael Jackson and the Wu-Tang Clan. You have given me the joy of hearing my daughter ask, 'Mummy, when can I have a meat dress?' before I've even had time to put the coffee on. You have given me the supportive, nourishing, kind, funny voices of my close friends, aka the Lady Family. You have given me the kind, patient, wise and thoughtful words of my mum and dad. When making documentaries you have given me the stories and experiences of the people who have opened up their lives to me. You have given me the energy and inspiration of the people I work with, who teach me, berate me, push me and lift me up after an eighteen-hour day and make me laugh when it's freezing cold and I really want a sausage roll and we've still got another eighteen hours to go.*

*Considering how often I abuse you, you deserve more than thanks. I have spent hours, years, at raves and gigs and festivals, standing stupidly close to the speakers and, even though you were ringing in pain afterwards, I ignored the alarm bell and did it again a week later. Ironically I didn't listen to my mum when she* told me I would go deaf if I kept pounding you with music; I didn't even consider at the time how devastating it would be to break you and I am pathetically grateful that I seem to have avoided that, I imagine pretty narrowly. Whilst I love loud music, it would not have been worth missing my son laughing to the point of hysteria as I poke his bum with a pencil.

The only time you have played up was when I pierced you at sixteen and you reacted in an angry and offended way, responding with a headache-inducing pus protest and vexed red swollen fury. But I think that, considering someone with questionable personal hygiene tried to stick a metal spike through you whilst being more concerned with refilling the incense burner, your reaction was justified. Even more so when I pierced you again and again, moving further upwards until I had run out of space and had to go inside, to the conch (which, until I just Googled it, I have always referred to as the 'insidey bit'). I did this when I was in Thailand (alarm bells) and the piercing salon was a hut on the beach that was shrewdly open at 1 a.m. for ravers to fulfil their impulses after several buckets of Thai rum and Thai Red Bull (which, I didn't realize at the time, allegedly contained a higher concentration of the wings-supplying ingredients than the UK version. That would explain why the period between 8 p.m. and 6 a.m. felt like twelve minutes). The piercing was done extremely slowly with a thick needle and felt like someone was removing you, one of my two beloved ears, from my head with a fork. That was not fun.

So, considering I have pumped near-deafening music into the depths of your weird-shaped curves and stabbed you with piercing guns and huge needles and have made you wear heavy earrings that

*my son likes to yank, you are a dream. I promise to look after you*
*better and to buy you a beautiful pair of earmuffs this winter and*
*to appreciate all the things you give me. For what is a life without*
*being able to listen to 'Man in the Mirror' every so often?*

## Music

My first musical eureka moment was thanks to Michael
Jackson. I was about six years old when I fell in love with
him. I listened to his album *Bad* so many times my whole
family ended up being able to mouth the words to every
song. I have so many fond memories of morning sing-a-
longs with my mum to 'Beat It' and, our other favourite,
'When a Man Loves a Woman' from Michael Bolton's
*Time, Love & Tenderness*, really giving it our all, followed by
Mick Hucknell's album *Stars*. The trip to school just wasn't
long enough.

My Saturday afternoons as a child were mostly spent
learning the moves to Michael Jackson music videos,
which was *fantastically* hard in those days as there was no
YouTube and no iTunes. All I could get my twitchy mitts
on was a VHS of his videos, which I would have to watch
in slow motion, press pause, copy the move, rewind and
repeat, again and again and again .... That is commitment.
And yet even though I have listened to his songs a hundred million times each, I still feel a thrill when someone
puts on 'Thriller'.

My next music lust was for De La Soul. I know that sounds extremely precocious but it was entirely accidental. I have three brothers and the eldest two are nearly a decade older than me. Whilst my third brother (eighteen months older than me) and I were busy eating hot Weetabix and golden syrup in our jim-jams and watching *The Raccoons*, my older brothers were doing cool, mysterious things like listening to records and going out (Where?! As a nine-year old I could not fathom where you could actually go, other than the playground or Wimpy). So one day, determined to find some common ground and gain an insight into these two shadowy figures in my life, I sneaked into their rooms and stole one thing that might tell me a little bit about them, which happened to be their De La Soul tape. Obviously I also had a really good snoop about but everything was so far removed from my world of Kylie and hair bobbles that it might as well have been in Klingon.

So off I trotted with my treasure – my first glimmer into the world of my older brothers. And the tape was clear – CLEAR! – which was mega. The first time I listened to it on my gigantic black stereo I thought it was a load of cobblers – what was with all the sort-of talking? Where were the backing singers? Where was the tear-inducing crescendo? Why weren't they singing about love? But because it was my only nugget of gold and because I was determined to like something my brothers liked, I turned it over and played side B. And then I played side A again and repeated this until I knew it off by heart. I still love it to this day.

My love of and need for music has never waned and I am always thirsty for more. At the moment I am in an R 'n' B place because I don't see nothing wrong with a little bump and grind. Most weekends my friend Amy and I, and whoever else we can bribe, make ourselves bulbous from nachos and vodka and then find somewhere, no matter how dank, to wind our bodeeez and wiggle our belleeez. It's hard to beat that combo – carbs, vodka and R. Kelly. I recently gave myself whiplash learning how to 'dutty wine' and have thighs of steel after mastering the 'slut drop', which is essentially Cossack dancing with a cross face.

## Listening

Listening to music is beautiful and simple and a joy. Listening to people is important and fascinating and complicated and sometimes very annoying. Sometimes I listen to people and I want to bonk them on the head. Sometimes they are listening to me and I suspect they want to bonk me on the head. Everyone loves music and animals as they never talk back and won't slam the door on their way out. That is why dogs are a man's best friend; yes, we have to pick up their extremely stinky poos and, yes, they cover the sofa in fur and, yes, sometimes they go into the garden, eat their own faeces and then lick the face of your child (my most recent encounter with a dog), but they are never passive aggressive or tell you home truths or make you feel guilt for not calling them back. However, they also can't wish you a happy birthday or know that when you say 'I'm fine' you might not be or stand up for you if people are talking behind your back. I do love dogs but I don't want them to be my best friends. I'm not entirely sure they'd enjoy slut-dropping with me to R. Kelly anyway.

As I've got older (and thus sexier and wiser and better dressed – I'll explain this later), I've realized that communicating with humans is unavoidable as I'm just not cut out for cave life. I get cold easily and I love microwaves and plumbing and fluffy towels that smell of Ocean Breeze. But, thankfully, I don't find human interaction vexing – I love it. I would rather be laughing and listening and being heard in a clapped-out Mini than being ignored in a Bentley. Humans and their humanness is everything, and the more human and flawed and frank the better.

As someone who interviews people for a living, I'm sure that isn't much of a surprise. I can listen to someone until the cows come home and even if they don't come home I'll sit there as long as someone wants to talk to me. I find people's stories fascinating and even the most 'boring' human being (no such thing really – it's more about how open and honest someone is) has layers and twists and turns if you dig deep enough. I feel lucky because my job provides an opportunity for people to tell me their deepest secrets within about five minutes of meeting me because they know that's why I am there and there is a sodding huge camera in their face. It's like going to a party and getting to the good bit without any periphery chat about house prices or anything else that is an (often very necessary) ice-breaking evil. So I arrive at their house after a producer has had a preliminary chat with them, we make tea and then off we go. And at the end of a ten-hour day they know everything about me and I know everything about them.

It is quite hard to then go to, say, a wedding where you can spend five hours with a group of people and know nothing more than where they live and what they do and what their cat is called. I am nosey and have been spoilt and want to know the innermost workings of everyone's being. Which just isn't appropriate in many settings.

As I've got older (and sexier and wiser and better dressed) I have realized that there are two types of listening: watching someone's mouth move whilst waiting for them to stop talking so you can make your next point, and concentrating on, and caring about, what someone is saying. The first doesn't really count as listening (and I'd like that to be a not-very-well-hidden message to a certain ex-boyfriend). The second is proper listening, and over the years I've learned a few more tricks:

## Breathe

I recently experienced couples therapy and found that sometimes it was so tense and stressful that I would forget to breathe. This would make me both turn slightly blue and become unable to think clearly. And, as a result, it would magnify the stress and make it impossible to react in a centred, calm way. It's also important to remember to breathe in the middle of an argument. There is no rush. Take your time. Give yourself room to think (I tell myself). As someone who very rarely fights (being more a flight-and-hide type), I tend to metaphorically curl up into a ball and hope that no one can see me and pray that it will all be over soon. I've done this since I was a little girl. If you're small and have no control over a scary situation, the most common reactions are to either learn how to become invisible and hope the threat won't be directed at you, or to become angry and hope that the threat will be deterred from coming to you. The extent to which you either retreat or fight is dependent on how severe the threat is. If the threat, be it parents or school or something else, is very big, then a child will respond accordingly. This continues into adulthood and is either something that a person lives with and has to manage or else spends a great deal of their disposable income trying to unpick and undo it in therapy. I have recently started personal therapy and unpicking is no small job. But I hope that, at the end of it, I will be able to have difficult, potentially confrontational conversations with people without feeling like the world is going to end.

OK, sorry, thank you for listening, back to listening and breathing. I have learned that if, during a difficult conversation, I remember to breathe (giving my brain oxygen and unclenching my chest and lungs to give my heart some space), I often automatically sit up straight rather than curling into myself, and I react in a much stronger, more adult, more honest way, and say what I mean rather than saying whatever I can to placate and thus end the fighting. I try to remind myself that when I'm in the mire of a fight I should pause. And breathe. And breathe again. And make myself pause and breathe as long as possible without adding any extra weirdness, so I can step away from the knee-jerk response. And I have learned most people are willing to wait for a moment, and are often thankful that the pace has been slowed as it also gives them a chance to breath and uncurl.

## Tune In

When I was little I used to think I was telepathic. This was mostly because whenever I went to a pantomime and they asked who would like to come on stage at the end I would *always* be picked. I was sure this was because I had stared into their eyes and was speaking into their brains. Looking back, it was probably something more to do with the fact that I was jumping up and down like I had Deep Heat on my bottom. (I did once put Deep Heat on my bottom at boarding school because I'd pulled a muscle and then, because the stinging was too much, pressed my naked butt cheeks against the only cold thing I could find – the window. We had a complaint from the old people's home next door about five minutes later and I felt a strange mixture of embarrassment and excitement at knowing that I would dine out on the story for years – and I was right).

So, of course I wasn't telepathic, but I was and am very, very sensitive. I sometimes walk into a room and know the people in there have been arguing (the blood on the wall can give it away). And, whilst I struggle with many, many things, this is something I am quite good at. I can hear the words coming out of people's mouths but I can also, sometimes, hear their feelings. Which seems even weirder written down than it does saying it. I know lots of people can do this and I'm sure those people also know it's both a blessing and a curse. I sometimes wish I could switch it off; when someone is quietly fuming or secretly despairing or invisibly distraught I can often feel it, even if it's a fun party where everyone is meant to be having a good time. This is essentially a very long-winded way of saying I have a strong sense of empathy and it's mostly a good thing and has sometimes been very useful. But I believe this is something that can be cultivated, almost like how a radio tunes in to different radio waves. A human being can tune themselves in to other humans if they want to. For some people their work is to develop their ability to tune in to people; for me, it's to learn how to sometimes tune out. Like giving myself a little emotional spa day. Sentences such as 'You are not responsible for how they react; you are only responsible for being kind and fair' and 'Their emotions are not your emotions' have been very helpful.

## Pick Your Battles

This is not technically a 'listening' lesson but definitely a highly valuable tip in managing relationships. I use this in every relationship I have, especially with my children where I use it so often it is worn through. And to offset my very long-winded paragraph on listening I'll keep this short and say that I've realized the importance of letting go of winning. It's not about point-scoring. It's not about proving you are right. Sometimes it's better to just back down, keep the peace, make sausages and watch *The Apprentice*.

## Eye Contact

This is very simple. If your eyes are darting around the room looking out for someone or something more fun to happen, this communicates only one message: *I'm not listening and I'm bored and I'm hoping something more fun will stop my brain from falling out of my ear*. This will not help you if you're trying to convince the person you're with that you're focused on them and care about what they're saying.

Looking at someone whilst listening to them is also one of the sexiest things a boy can do to a girl – it makes her feel cherished and sexy – and vice versa. (Warning, another dig at an ex-boyfriend: staring at a hot girl sitting on a stool at the bar in a short skirt is *not* affirming or helpful and makes the girl you're with feel like an invisible piece of crap. Oh, and the excuse that you're looking at her boobs because she has really pointy nipples does not help the situation. I'm sorry, that was a very direct dig and I think it didn't even massively relate to the point. Moving on.)

## Mirror It

This is something very therapy-ish but at times of real conflict I think it works. If you find that you're going around and around the same point and you want to beat the other person to a pulp because they don't seem to be hearing you, ask them to tell you their point and then calmly repeat what they say. If you can both agree, in the moment, what has been said, it reduces the chance of anyone being able to twist it later. Alternatively ask them to write it down and, if you don't like it, you can dramatically burn it to ash whilst walking away (cue sexy music). Also, if you still find that you are not hearing each other, having a third party to help you do the hearing (therapist/ trusted friend) can be a relationship saver.

## Stall

If all else fails, stall. Use the sentence 'Hmm, how interesting, let me ponder upon that' or, if you're not from the 1920s, you could say, 'Hang tight, I need some time to think about that.' This gives everyone a cooling-off period and you (well, me) time to Google any words or references you didn't understand and to think about how you'd like to reply. It also stops heat-of-the-moment responses such as, 'Yeah, well, you smell like poo!' and 'Kiss your mama with that mouth?' Both great, but not massively productive.

The art of communication is one of the most important parts of a relationship. But it's also one of the hardest. So sometimes it's important just to keep shtum.

## Silence

I'm pretty sure that the ability to sit in silence and listen to the still, small voice inside yourself is one of the keys to a happy life, but I think it also happens to be one of the hardest things to do in the whole entire world – even worse than surfing, which is freakishly hard, or walking up a non-moving escalator without commenting on how weird it feels.

I recently went through a very painful, complicated situation and at the time I felt emotionally wretched. I started personal therapy, having thought it would be a waste of money (I used to think that I didn't need therapy because I have lovely friends – but I now see that therapy is very different from chatting over a bowl of pasta in someone's kitchen), and I now think therapy is brilliant. I love and value the sessions and realize that a therapist can challenge and guide and illuminate and draw hidden things out in a way that even the closest, most astute friend can't do. Each therapy session has been fantastically helpful and enlightening in a way I could not have predicted. I know that since I have been doing it I've started to understand myself, I am a better parent and I'm a better friend. Some people say it is selfish to spend money on therapy for yourself but I think it is a kindness to others.

So, back to the hideous soul-and-mind-scrambling life dilemma. In a bid to try to help me work out what to do, many people told me to listen to the still, small voice inside myself. Well, gosh, that sounds so simple! Brilliant! The answer is within! But whereas years ago I had the experience of being in a peaceful place where I was able to connect with this part of myself, I most certainly am not now. With a busy, unpredictable job, two lovely nutter kids, a toing-and-froing city life, lists lists lists, a phone, music, texts, Instagram, Facebook, Twitter and about a hundred different people's opinions on my situation whirling around my noggin, the chance of being able to hear that very small but very poignant voice is non-existent.

I am currently in the process of trying to rediscover it. Like turning on the unflattering lights at the end of a rave and emptying out an overcrowded room, I need to gradually push out the noise and chatter and busyness. I know that the more time I invest in being quiet and turning off my phone, the closer I will be to understanding how I truly feel about my situation. But, God, that is so much harder than it sounds.

And I think that's *exactly* why I *do* fill my life and my airwaves with distractions. I run away from silence because that is where I feel real emotion. That is the moment when I stop looking at what everyone *else* is doing (Twitter, etc.) and start to look at how *I* am doing. And because the feelings I avoid and push away are often fear and sadness, when I stop and sit still, those are the ones that hit me in the face. Which reconfirms to me the importance of never sitting still and never being quiet and never turning off my phone for more than a few minutes because then I might actually have those feelings.

But what I forget is that when I just sit with it and ride it out and wait for the initial brain-panic to slow down, it *will* eventually stop, and on the other side is sometimes happiness, sometimes balance and sometimes peace. Sometimes all three.

I am kicking myself as I write this because I have been doing *everything* possible to avoid feeling sad and scared – my house looks like a hotel at the moment and my toenails are neat and the jams are aligned in my fridge. Please send help. I'm frustrated because five minutes is such a very short time to spend doing something that makes me so happy and healthy. I exercise most days and I eat my greens and I brush my hair (sometimes) and take multivitamins. But when it comes to doing something that has such a positive impact on my mental and emotional well-being, I just don't make the time. Which is bonkers as I always feel lighter and calmer and happier as a result.

In fact, I should probably go and practise sitting in silence right now. But I'm not going to because – *quick, quick, Brain, think of SOMETHING!* – I'm writing this chapter, and oh, look, I've got a new text, and a really great song has just come on, and I must immediately re-do my hair right this minute. So I'll do it tomorrow. Yeah. Defo.

I'm aware of the huge value in being quiet. But, as I can't yet endure total silence and stillness, I often opt for the nursery slopes: a café. For some people their thinky place is when they are running or in the shower or swimming or doing a poo. For me it's cafés. It's the environment where I find it easiest to relax, to think, to understand my thoughts, to come to terms with difficult feelings, to evaluate, process, realign and breathe (and drink coffee). It's not as good as being somewhere totally quiet and still, but baby steps. Whilst being at home is lovely and fun, it's not somewhere I can completely let my mind wander, as there is always laundry to be done or nooks to be tidied or food that could be prepared or cleared up.

The other time I am at my most lucid is with my friends. Another important function of ears is that they are an external processor. I sometimes have to *hear* myself saying something in order to understand my feelings about it. I don't know how many times I've been jabbering on about something to a friend and during the conversation had a revelation. *Oh. Oh, I see. This is because of X and Y and Z. HOW have I not seen that before?*

And so it's back to the importance of caring, focused listening. Because my patient friends understand me and let me jabber on (within reason), they give me the gift of time and the opportunity to organize my floating thoughts into solid sentences that follow on from each other, which almost always results in a solution or plan of action (and this is almost always celebrated with a Hobnob or a glass of wine depending on what time of day it is). Good friends that you have a full-disclosure policy with are as valuable to your health as your local GP. In fact, that 'full-disclosure' part is, I've realized, *incredibly* important and something I think is very precious and quite rare. If you have friends like that, hang on to them for dear life. If there are a few people whose judgement you trust (the more the merrier) in your life, who you can be a hundred per cent honest with, no matter how mean or grimey or awful your thoughts and feelings are, then you allow yourself to be challenged and advised and therefore you allow yourself to grow. If you are always editing what you say and consciously pres- enting yourself in a particular way, you will both never develop and never have that wonderful, wonderful feeling of being fully known and fully accepted. Plus your friends will never be able to tease you and that is no fun.

## Negative Voices

So, whilst I've learned (well, am learning) how important it is to listen to yourself and others carefully and regularly, there is *one* voice it's important to COMPLETELY IGNORE.

And that's the voice inside us telling us we're shit, which tells us people think we're stupid, arrogant, fat, wearing a ridiculous outfit, undeserving, not a good mother, not good at our job, not at the cool party, have crap hair (these are all things I've thought this week). It's the critical voice that never goes away, that we *must* learn to shout over and put back in its box. It is the little gremlin that can ruin a joyous evening by telling you that you've put on weight and look ridiculous in your leather trousers, or that feeds your insecurity by telling you that other people are doing better than you and so you might as well not bother.

That whispering toxic gremlin must be identified and vanquished as though you were swatting an irritating mosquito on holiday. Just squash it. Tell it to sod off, that you are far too busy to hear that shit. It's unhelpful and unconstructive. Off you trot.

A friend of mine who runs a fairly big business, the same as mentioned earlier, told me how he observed that, unfailingly, when it came to performance reviews, the men told him they were brilliant and deserved a promotion and a pay rise and the women (even the senior ones) told him about areas they needed to develop. So, whilst the idea of squashing this voice is lovely, how do we *really* stop ourselves from paying heed to the gremlin? I think there are four things:

### Good friendships

I can't count the amount of times I have opened up about my work or relationship or physical insecurity and been easily and quickly comforted back to goodness by a friend.

### Knowing yourself

Which means listening to yourself and taking the time to be quiet. In this process you can learn what your gremlin-triggers are (in my case, being around other mums who seem to effortlessly juggle their healthy organic lives and have glossy hair, or being around people without children who can go out as late as they want or work as long as they want and recover with a delicious lie-in the next day rather than being woken up at 7 a.m. by a very cute but very hungry person, or other telly people that seem to be cooler and more successful than me). I now know that sometimes these things make me feel bad about myself so I keep an eye on it. This way you can catch the gremlin before it's even woken up.

### Growing older

One of the best things about getting older is that, because you have been practising points 1) and 2), it becomes easier to spot when the gremlin is on the warpath and to squish it with one KERSPLAT.

### Defiance

This is when you simply decide not to care. Grab not-caring by the balls and wang it around like you just don't care. Put on not-caring like you are adorning yourself with a beautiful robe. Just decide to not care if you don't look 'perfect' (which doesn't really exist) or like the glossy girl in the magazine or like the yoga puma on Instagram; just decide to appreciate them – enjoy them whilst also appreciating and loving yourself. *Remember* to love yourself. Give yourself permission to be happy and to feel good about yourself. I sometimes think we feel bad for loving ourselves – like we're worried it will lead to arrogance. But it won't. It will probably just lead to you having a better day. And we only get 365 of those a year so we might as well make the most of them.

I would love my daughter to have such a strong sense of self and such good self-esteem that she doesn't have to battle against a gremlin, but I have yet to meet a woman or man who is totally free of one. So, in light of that, I hope she surrounds herself with nourishing, wise friends. Because it's in the mire of human interaction that we really learn and grow and feel good and feel alive. It's the chemical, fleshy, lovely, smelly, real human beings having a cup of tea, or another glass of wine, eyeball to eyeball, because that white-of-the-eye interaction that makes us feel whole and loved and happy. It can't happen on Twitter. It can't happen on a mobile phone. It can't happen with a Facebook 'like'. And whilst I *love* social media (I am that heinous person taking a photograph of my croissant to post on Instagram and feeling both shame and the strange compulsion to do it regardless), I do think it's a hindrance to silence and calm and humanness, and it can be like a feeding tube directly into the stomach of our little grizzly gremlins.

I run the risk of sounding like a granny and I should probably start using the word 'interweb', but I do think our generation is only now working out what the internet giveth and what it taketh away. It acts as an easy and never-ending distraction from listening to ourselves; it prevents us from properly listening to others and it feeds our negative gremlin. It has expanded our reach and our understanding of each other and it's *really* fun, but I think we are only now just working out how to ingest it in a healthy way. Like a starving kid in a sweet shop, we have gorged ourselves on Kim's bum, bloggers' fave pix, on weekend getaways that we weren't invited to, on inspirational quotes and cats in sausage hats and great shoes and conspiracy theories and political campaigns and cats in cake hats and swiping right and left and Kim's boobs and cats in potato hats . . . but thankfully we are starting to realize the importance of disconnecting from the digital world and engaging in the three-dimensional world – because the antidote to the negative impact of the interweb is those lovely, confusing, comforting, listening and responding human beings. This most definitely leads on to what the internet/porn has done to people's expectations/enjoyment of sex BUT that is a big fish to fry and I shall return to that later with great excitement and horn.

It is also always comforting to be with a real human in the present moment when they are having a nice time rather than seeing their Instagram pictures from when they were having The Best Time Ever and, thanks to filters, look all ethereal and beautiful like they've just stepped out of a Wes Anderson film. It's good to remind ourselves that, even at Coachella (surely the worst offender for causing intense FOMO), people have to queue for Portaloos. I sometimes worry about the effect my Instagram has on others. Whilst it is far from glossy and there is no hint of a trip to the Maldives or flowing chiffon (a nightmare on the school run), it doesn't really communicate my real experience of everyday life. At no point would anyone, if they looked at my picture history, think I've been feeling anything other than love for my children, happiness at work or fun with my friends. You would not be able to see, even if you looked really hard and really long, any hint of tension in relationships, arguments, worry about money, guilt about being a working mum, anxiety about the future or self-criticism. And whilst I'm not saying that it's easy or realistic to post a picture every time you forget to send your kids to school with the right PE kit, I do think it's important to remind each other, often, of how very, very curated most social media is.

Which brings me back to the point that the internet is very powerful and very fun but that Actual Real Humans with context and stories and emotions you can feel and question are far more empowering, encouraging and trustworthy – they are the bee's knees.

# Unhelpful Things to Hear

I just want to take a quick minute to mention something that I feel is an epidemic at the moment and very unhelpful: Rubbish Modern Sayings. They are bandied about, often on prime-time television, because they sound nice and are easy to say and make people cry. However, when you think about them for five minutes they don't make any sense and aren't very helpful:

## Believe in Your Dreams and They Will Come True

This is the king of rubbish sayings. If you work hard and put yourself in the right place and turn up on time and love what you do and answer emails quickly and be polite, not just for a week but again and again, you'll gradually move closer to what you dream of. But it doesn't matter how hard you believe something or how beautiful your dreams are, if you hit the snooze button in the morning it's not going to happen.

## It's Political Correctness Gone Mad

It is very, very rare for someone to be careful about not offending someone or sensitive about how they're referring to people and for it not to be a completely great and kind and sane thing to do.

## People Should Just Accept Me for Who I Am

But what if you're being a proper plonker? The joy of friends is that they both love you *and* have an outside view of you and, if done gently and with the motive of helping rather than hurting you, feedback can be incredibly, life-changingly useful. But you have to be open to it. I personally believe that we should be constantly changing, especially our pants but also our habits.

## It's the Thought That Counts

No it's not. It's the action. If you're thinking about calling a friend who isn't having a nice time but you never actually do it, does that person feel loved? If you think about buying someone a thank-you present but don't do it, does that person feel appreciated? I learned this a few years ago when I *really meant* to call a friend who was going through a divorce and I thought about her a lot but I never actually did anything because I was being lazy and I told myself I was busy, but really I just hadn't prioritized. And it made me realize that the thought only counts if it's followed by action. I have to remind myself of this frustratingly often.

## The Best Things Come to Those Who Wait

Nope. Things come to those that get on with it. Or as I like to say: people who Get Shit Done.

OK, now for something more fun.

I am always learning, often by making mistakes, about how important it is to communicate well in a relationship about feelings and logistics and care and compassion. And I am also aware of the importance of communicating rude and naughty things that make your bits hot or, as my friend Sam says, get fizzy knickers. Yes, it's sexy talk.

I am finding this part very hard to write as, in the cold light of day when it's raining outside and I'm in a baggy jumper and bad pants, it's INSANELY awkward to talk about. It's actually one of those things that is best left unsaid unless right in the moment, but for the purposes of this book I am going to break that rule.

Firstly, talking dirty is massively, hugely underrated. When done well it's like throwing a very hot grenade into your sex life. However, for many people it's just too weird and too awkward and, for the most part, I fall into that category. But at the same time I am a huge advocate of life being very short and just giving it a whirl.

This is one of the few subjects I recently realized I haven't talked about with my friends. It is so deeply personal. And when I posed it as a subject the other night and asked how they felt about it and how they did it, we spent most of the time laughing until snot came out of our noses. I highly recommend asking your friends to repeat the kinds of things they say in the heat of the moment because it is really, really funny. You might also be surprised, as I was, when you discover what they have been texting to their lovers. It's always the quiet ones.

We did manage to stop snotting for long enough to formulate some golden dirty-talk tips and tricks. List time again!

1. Always gently assess how comfortable the other person is – this is a game best played with a willing partner. If you scream *'Ride me like a donkey at the beach!'* without having built it up slowly, then you are in danger of never hearing from that person again.

2. Dirty talk is only hot if there is no embarrassment, so, whilst treading carefully at first, once you're sure it's being received well go for it with conviction. A G & T or five don't hurt to break the ice. Never say 'um' or 'er' phrases, such as *'No, hang on, I take that back'* or *'What's the word I'm thinking of? It rhymes with list'*.

3. This is one of the few things that you can't really practise. Hence the importance of starting gently and building up. Although I would highly recommend trying out a few phrases with your friends if you want a bloody good laugh.

4. One of the best ways to introduce smutty chat into your relationship is via text. Not only can you take your time and compose the first few carefully but you can also assess the response in your own time and, if you're nervous about

stepping into this arena, perhaps even show your most trusted friends to make sure your reply isn't crackers or something that will land you in prison.

5. Never *ever* laugh. Even if they have said something utterly, brain-twistingly obscure, hold the giggle in. In all other instances in a relationship laughter is beautiful and bonding and important, but when it comes to dirty talk try to stay in the moment. If it really is something that made an impression, perhaps gently address it afterwards in a very delicate way. I have one friend who, in a bid to conceal the giggles, ended up shaking with her entire body, which translated into an orgasm that benefited both of them and saved the other person's feelings. Bonza.

6. Whilst guffawing with laughter mid-bonking session is not advised, feedback afterwards is definitely a good idea. That is much harder than it sounds but worth doing (perhaps after a few tequila shots) as it's a win-win.

It's worth noting that I am aware that for most people under the age of twenty-five, having grown up with the internet and porn and mobiles and texting and sexting, the idea that you would take sexting advice from a thirty-four-year-old woman is hysterically funny. If that is the case then I am glad that at the very least I have provided you with an insight into what it's like to be an adult and still getting to grips with this sex tech thingy.

# 9. Letter to My Bum: Size, Bum Admin, The Face of Bum

*'Sup, Bum,*

*Whilst I have had to apologize to my fanny for a lack of attention, I have to apologize to you for too much attention. My disclaimer is that I've grown up in the Kate Moss era, when having anything more rounded and soft than an ironing board was considered unsightly and, well, gross. If you had your way, you would be two rotund comfortable cheery cheeks, but at the insecure and trend-aware age of sixteen, I decided that I would beat you into submission. There wasn't one girl or woman in any of the magazines who had anything resembling a bottom like mine. The message I took from this was that my bottom was an embarrassing design mistake.*

*So, instead of letting you be, I have squatted, lunged and burpee'd you in the hope that you will defy gravity. Not that you haven't put up a fight, which I now respect, but at the time I cursed you for not fitting into a pair of skinny jeans without cutting off the blood supply to the rest of my body. But, you may have noticed, I am now on your side. I am starting to enjoy your cushiony goodness and am trying to treat you better. I hope you've appreciated my recent rejection of clothes that make you uncomfortable; I have binned my gigantic beige Spanx with their special little wee hole (always great for making a woman feel glamorous and full of love) and I am consciously starting to accept and love your natural shape and texture.*

*I see now that not only are you a cushion but you are also a wonderful part of being a woman. And that is nothing to hide or try to prevent or be ashamed of. A bottom, a bottomy bottom, with curvy curves and squeeziness and even, Good God, dimples, is delicious.*

*And now, when I look at you in the mirror, I forcefully tell myself, 'I am not a nine-year-old boy. It's OK that I have a pair of round pinchable cheeks. They are there for a reason and that reason is comfort and joy and sexiness made flesh.' I am a woman that has softness and curves and bits that wobble and move sometimes with only the slightest of breezes. I promise that I will never again suffocate you in a pair of spray-on-tight jeans or underwear that cuts you into four sections like a joint of beef about to be roasted.*

*This is phase two of our relationship and I will make every effort to liberate you, appreciate you and enjoy you. But it takes a long time to retrain a brain and after thirty-odd years of observing only tiny rock-hard bottoms in the media, you'll have to bear with me – I will get there. In the meantime, this quote is for you: 'There is nothing as overrated as bad sex and nothing as underrated as a good poo.'*

## Size

So, let's start with the facts. Women generally have bigger bums than men because we are extremely sensible and have evolved to have a built-in cushion – well, OK, really because we've evolved to store fat there to help grow babies. That, and the fact that we need a bigger pelvis so that it's really easy and comfortable for a baby to come out of our love tunnels. You may detect just a tiny, weeny hint of sarcasm – take note, Mother Nature: your work here is not done. Our pelvises also tend to tilt backwards and therefore make our derrières protrude more than men's. And until recently there was a strong cultural belief that women with bigger backsides had healthier children. It was survival of the fullest.

But I am delighted that during my adult years I have witnessed a shift from the nineties, when predominately teeny bottoms adorned the fashion pages, to the noughties when we saw something of an explosive appreciation for the gluteus maximus. I'd like to take this opportunity to give my thanks to J-Lo, Beyoncé, Nicki Minaj and Kim Kardashian – they are tail trailblazers.

I was recently shopping for lingerie (which has become significantly more enjoyable now I have started to embrace, both metaphorically and literally, my squeezy cheekies) and was admiring the smoking-hot body of the girl serving me. She had big boobs, a big bum and a big warm smile. She was gorgeous. As we mused on needing an engineering PhD to find good underwear, she said how much she hated her 'short fat body'. I hated to hear her say that but I wasn't surprised. Even though, to me and anyone with eyes, she was off-the-scale sexy, I could absolutely see why she didn't feel she had a 'good' body. As ladies of roughly the same age, it's not hard to imagine that we had been equally bombarded with images of willowy, ethereal racehorses. Obvs I told her she was smoking hot but I could tell she didn't believe me – what's one comment against two decades of absorbing the message that less is more?

However wonderful it is that larger buttocks are back in fashion, I suspect it is really just another trend and will therefore fade when the next one takes over (which will probably be adoration of people with massive thumbs). I know it's part of the fashion industry and I know that this industry is hugely important and gives people employment, but it vexes me that women's bodies are subject to trends.

Of course it all depends on whether you buy into what is trendy or whether you are immune to changing fashion trends and, whilst occasionally I march to the beat of my own drum, I am mostly a total sucker for fast fashion. I am the person that buys the Day-Glo maxi skirt and wears it with purple clogs for exactly one whole month before I realize that only Alexa Chung can pull this 'look' off and perhaps it's time to stop looking like an Austrian pensioner milkmaid.

And so, in the same way, I am subconsciously affected (frustratingly) by what body type is in fashion. And I feel confident in saying that I am not alone in this. Otherwise the magazines that ridicule women's bodies for being anything other than the accepted shapes would be bankrupt and their employees would have to use their journalistic and photographic talents for something other than shaming women.

I have always envied those girls (I have met perhaps only one or two in my lifetime, but thanks to the glory of Instagram I am nurtured by them on a regular basis) who wear whatever they like, be it stripy socks or skintight green sequined fishtail dresses with nautical hats and pink eyeshadow and rainbow hairbands, because they seem so free from what is dictated by 'fashion'. (Incidentally I don't mean to anthropomorphize fashion into some awful wicked monster that hates women, but I do think we need to reclaim it and shove it back into a healthy and happy place.) I always wonder how these women got there. How did they get to the place where they backcomb their hair into a brilliant giant beehive and stick a giant neon-yellow bow into it and slick on some shimmery purple eyeshadow and don't give a fuck if a boy thinks that is sexy or whether it is trendy or chic or socially acceptable but just do it because they wanted to? Was it conscious? Did they all listen to the same TED Talk? Did they all go to the same school of Not Giving A Fuck? I'll have what they're having.

These women who have open, free expression have had a huge impact on me. And whilst there are many things more lofty to concern ourselves with than the clothes on our backs, they are, for many people, a daily way to creatively express ourselves. Sadly there is a kind of dictatorship about what is Right and what is Wrong and many of us are not immune to it. Fashion should be an arena to be playful in; it should be joyful. Yet often it's not – the slick highly styled not-a-hair-out-of-place look that is favoured by the majority of magazines is beautiful to look at but it's way beyond the reach of most of us mere mortals. Today I flicked through a magazine stand and found approximately twelve articles devoted to the flawless, sartorially totalitarian style of Olivia Palermo. I wish there was equal celebration and coverage of those real, imperfect, inspirational human beings who choose to display their incredible creativity through clothes.

Walking the red carpet, often viewed as a glamorous and fun event, is actually a bit of a bloody nightmare. It has a smattering of walking the plank about it. It terrifies me. I get the same feeling as I do before a huge exam. And that's because it *is* a huge exam. It's a test of how many green juices you consumed in the three months beforehand; it's a test of how many PT sessions you've made it to at 5 a.m.; and of whether you got the memo on what is the right thing to wear at that particular moment in fashion history. And God help you if they get a photo from behind and you haven't spent the previous six weeks squatting like a Russian dancer on speed. From my few experiences of doing it, I understand why so many actresses dread it and play it extremely safe in an extremely classic gown with extremely tidy hair. I'd secretly love to know what Kate Middleton would actually wear if she wasn't subject to such close inspection – I think if she wore a matching rainbow cropped T-shirt and skirt with her hair in a skull-top bun the world might actually explode.

Of course there is a place in the wide world of fashion for every flavour. But I am so grateful for the carefree, liberated attitude some girls have towards their bodies and fashion. When I see these free people flash up on my Instagram feed I immediately feel a pressure lift. I shouldn't need it but it's like these women give me permission to not be beholden to the rules. Some things are infectious and this is certainly one of them. I'm not naturally, and will never be, someone who massively experiments with style, but I love that I am exposed to those who are free enough to do so every time I have a little scroll. It's social media at it's best. Thank you to those carefree women. Long live your presence on Instagram. You are a rare breed. You are a breath of fresh air.

Ten years ago, and often now, if you are willowy and look a little like you are on heroin you were/are bang on trend. Now it's also OK to have a bottom so big that you can balance a glass of champagne on it. Anything in between is just sooooo not OK. It sometimes feels that a woman's physical self, and therefore sadly her self-esteem, is a game of Russian roulette. Someone, probably living in a castle and stroking a white cat in a swingy chair, is deciding what these 'So Hot Right Now' bodies are.

Hey, maybe, like, stop it? Maybe go and make yourself a sandwich and decide what else your wonderful brain can contribute to the planet. Maybe don't spend your short, precious time on this earth making women feel crap for cash. Maybe stop writing mean articles about normal attractive women '*pouring*' or '*squeezing*' themselves into their outfits when what you're really saying is that they are FAT and GROSS and that they should go home.

So many women's magazines' primary function seems to be to shame other women – it's so gladiatorial. And *millions* of women compulsively read these articles, often secretly and with embarrassment, myself included. They are so addictive and seem to scratch an itch deep within our not-best self. And sadly, not only do we confirm to the magazine market that these articles sell, we also sub-consciously absorb the message that our bodies are ugly and disgusting unless they resemble a Victoria's Secret angel. It's a bit of a shmeggy, vicious, unhelpful – but lucrative – circle.

Of course some women read this stuff and think, *What a bunch of arse*, but they're lucky and, sadly, rare. For many, many years I was in the oh-shit-I-look-like-her-and-they're-saying-she-is-disgusting-so-I-must-be camp. I'm glad, for me, that that ship has sailed (or is at least out of the dock), but in the twenty-first century it is utterly lame that it's still happening. Some magazines and papers regu-larly publish articles about the damaging, degrading effects of porn on women today, but their own equally toxic, albeit much stealthier, 'journalism' is no less abusive. This is the age of commercial space flight, mass-produced electric sports cars and non-invasive laser surgery; surely we should be able to move on from telling women that their perfectly strong and healthy thighs are really yucky.

So I am glad that the new-wave big-bottom trend is on the rise. I hope it rises like a phoenix out of the ashes in a glory of trumpets and angels rejoicing and stays there, and I hope that whoever invented skinny jeans is forced to eternally watch a video of a woman giving birth to remind them that we are the creators and carriers and feeders of new human life and we really *need* two lovely big butt cheeks to make this happen. Which is, I reckon, probably quite important.

## Bum Admin

I'd never given any thought to bum admin until this year when I realized that it's 'a thing'. In fact, until two years ago when I made a programme that looked at hair 'management' (i.e. the amount of time women spend on waxing, cutting, colouring, styling, etc.), I had never given much thought to whether I found any of this beautifying vexing or not. I just did it. I knew, or felt, that it was wrong to be hairy, that all women should be briefed that if you venture outside with hairy legs, an anti-hair team would immediately arrest you and send you to work in a coal mine in Siberia.

So, as a good citizen, I dealt with my disgusting hair. But after thinking about it for more than four minutes I realized that this wasn't something I had chosen to do; it was something I did out of fear of being a social outcast. I met some amazing women who had bucked the trend of removing their hair, and even tried it for myself. Eventually, though, I returned to being hair-free – and it's impossible to know whether I did this because it was a genuine personal choice or because I bowed to the pressure of conformity. Whatever the reasons, I do think it's important to keep talking about this and examining it. It would be lovely, one day, for women to know that what they are doing is because of a genuine personal preference rather than because they are subconsciously picking up societal expectations and fear of being sent back from whence they came.

This was when I started to reflect upon the other bits of body admin that I undertook without thinking. And I realized that my bum also has a list of management requirements. As previously mentioned, it has been subjected to exercise, which I don't really mind as a) I enjoy it, b) I am like a dog and need walking every day, and c) it makes me feel good to be strong so that I can carry my kids and shopping and fight Bruce Lee. But apparently this is *far* from sufficient. I am now expected to buff it, massage it, tan it, have special cellulite and firming cream for it and, God help me, wax and bleach my bum hole. Yes, even the hair that you can't see unless you are a yogic giraffe has to be removed and the surrounding area 'prettied up'.

OK. Just hang tight for a moment. I need a second to scream into my armpit. Are you freaking kidding me?

Is it not enough that we rip out our sensitive pubic hair? Hair that is there to protect our fanny from a plethora of nasties, hence the dramatic rise in genital warts since the start of the Brazilian trend. Thank you, porn, always a friend to us.

So, now that we have plucked, buffed, creamed, squatted and adorned our bum in an uncomfortable but sexy G-string that rides up our crack all day, we can move on to something fun: PORN!

I say 'FUN' but really, how fun is it? Watching porn is a bit like eating too many Haribo. It gives delight and pleasure in the short term and then your teeth go all furry and you eventually slump into a sugar coma. OK, porn and Haribo aren't that similar. But stay with me.

Yes, watching porn is hot and yes I have done it. I have explored various categories and experienced the entire rainbow of reactions from bliss to terror. But, as I now realize, it is the main source of sexual education for teenagers, compared to the slightly more tame days when I was learning about sex from trial and error, and I feel a bit worried about how that is going to affect their perspective on what a girl/boy wants, what a girl/boy should look like and what it looks like to connect with the person they are having sex with. If porn is anything to go by, emotional connection is as far from the minds of the participants as whether they should give their granny a call. However, in my experience, the strength of the emotional connection is what takes sex from good to amazing. So much has been written about the effects of porn today on young people – and the general conclusion is that it is harmful. Sex in porn is fast, furious and often requires the woman to be a human sex toy that is programmed to moan loudly for the whole nine minutes it lasts. She should also be entirely hairless with the physique of a Barbie. It also normalizes sexual exercises that not everyone is comfortable with. For example, violent blow jobs or anal sex might be amazingly sexy for some, for others it's not. But in Porn Land it is the norm. And so, if you are a teenage boy or girl trawling through the hundreds of porn videos available, you might start to think it is the Done Thing. And that if you aren't a fan, you are a bit weird. So what would I do? Well, I think if I was a teenager with that example of sex in front of me, I would follow suit, whether I was comfortable with it or not. Because, remembering what it feels like to be a teenager, not fitting in was something to avoid at all costs. It's such a strange time as you're separating from your parents and the security of your childhood comforts, which means the need to be accepted by your friends/tribe is survival-strong. I remember doing everything to distinguish myself from my parents and doing whatever my friends were doing.

The shining light in this rather depressing state of affairs is the new movement towards producing responsible porn. It was previously called Porn for Women but, surely, this more consciously made porn is for everyone? Porn is, without a doubt, hot and we've been doing it ever since we could make art. Just go to the British Library and look at the Greek pots; they are absolutely covered in it. Humans like watching other humans having sex. It's fun. And I love that there are clever people now making porn that tries to depict a scenario where everyone involved is having a good time, rather than a scenario where one person is having a good time and the other person is just there. It's another healthy choice about what to feed ourselves.

## The Face of Bum

What better way to end a chapter about bums than to talk about my career high, perhaps life high, in being the Face of Bum in America.

My career has taken me on a lot of adventures, such as riding a man dressed like a horse and witnessing a home birth, but this has been one of the most unexpected. I vividly remember when I received the phone call from my agent telling me the news. I was filming a consumer programme and was at a sofa factory trying not to fall asleep on the job whilst delivering a piece to camera on perhaps the world's softest chaise longue. I called her back during a coffee (double espresso) break and she explained that an American brand was interested in my fronting a campaign for adult bum wipes. True. Of course I was nervous at first but the fee was great and the creative content was very funny. Before any decisions were made, the brand wanted to check I was open enough to discuss embarrassing topics and so we organized a Skype call for later that week. And I'm fairly confident that they had no question about whether I was OK talking about poo after that conversation. And just for good measure, I threw in some chat about piles to really seal the deal. I was born for the job.

We filmed the adverts in Los Angeles and they involved me running around asking complete strangers how they wiped their bums. And because the creative agency are a total hoot, they chose venues with excellent pun potential – for example, a bowling alley (up your alley, I thank you), a car show (how do you clean your bumper? I thank you) and an airport (the runway is clear, I thank you). And after being nervous about the potential embarrassment and critical response to making a loo-paper advert I can say, with relief, they were great. This is entirely down to the extremely brave brand who decided to veer away from using a cuddly bear to sell toilet paper, the brilliant PR team and creative team who had complete confidence in the idea and the amazing director who is nothing short of utterly bonkers.

I suggested that they could put my face on the sheets of paper but, for some reason, they declined. My legacy will have to be something else.

# The Conclusion *Big Loud Kettle Drums Booming*

... OR the Final Ramblings of a delirious person who has reached the end of a marathon and hadn't realized how long it was and isn't even sure why they ran it in the first place, but they have bleeding nipples and chaffing between the thighs so it's not all bad. Enjoy!

I don't know how I would feel if I was reading a book where the author admitted that one of their personal motos is 'The more I know, the more I realize I don't know very much'.

When I was little I assumed that grown-ups knew it all, and that when I was really, really old, say in my thirties, I would be fantastically wise and knowledgeable and would definitely know the capital of the Philippines and where the 1968 Summer Olympics were held (I Googled it, it was Mexico FYI) and other vital information. I took it for granted that I would be able to navigate life with swan-like grace and sometimes children would gather round a campfire to hear my stories of yore.

Now I am thirty-five I realize that only one part of this vision is true. I am handling it like a swan; it seems relatively smooth on the surface but underneath I am paddling like a loon. And, whilst the paddling has definitely become less random and more considered as I've gathered some degree of wisdom, the challenges have become bigger and in some cases the stakes are so life-changingly high, and affect other people in such an acute way, it almost feels too big to grasp. There have been some decisions that are so big it has felt like my brain has left my body in protest about having to make such a huge choice, leaving my stomach and my heart looking at each other, scratching their heads and wondering what the hell to do.

Over the years, things I felt absolutely certain about, like Take That being together for ever, don't seem too solid now. Promises I made (*I will love you for ever, Marky Mark*), passions I felt, views and beliefs I thought to be true, have all changed or at the very least shifted. The more I experience, the more I question and the more the world, well, my perspective, changes. That feels both unnerving and exciting. But that also makes me nervous about committing anything to paper, as I'm very much a work in progress. But I told myself when I had writer's block after writing four words and freaking out, if no one shared anything until they were a hundred per cent certain that they were correct then we would probably have a grand total of ten books and several of them would be about jam.

So what's my point? you are certainly and validly asking, especially now I've admitted how little I know. Well, my point is that, whilst we have an ever-increasing snow-storm of information and images constantly swirling in and out of our eyes and ears and brains and hearts, it's even more important to be as honest as possible with each other, even if we get it wrong sometimes. Because, whilst technology is changing so quickly it makes me feel about 200 years old just looking at the App Store, some things never change. Like wanting to feel included, loved, relevant and understood. And I think that happens when we're seeing and hearing the real experience of other people's lives. When I encounter something that feels real (i.e. anything written by Caitlin Moran and any Mothers Meeting event) it is so reassuring – it's a human connecting in a real, almost secret, way with another. It breaks down the barriers between us and makes us feel known and not alone. I love the new wave of female writers sharing their experiences of being a woman and working and relationships and parenting – sometimes lonely, sometimes not, sometimes happy, sometimes not, beautiful, scary, imperfect life-wrangling. These books, articles, tweets and Instagrams are like the ultimate anti-Photoshop medication; the internet on a good hair day.

Short of locking our children up in a cupboard (again, I've Googled it and it's really illegal) there isn't a way of entirely protecting them from all the dangers of the world. And there is no book or podcast or app that gives a foolproof way to ensure that they have a happy, fulfilling and authentic life. But I've realized what I can do is try to teach my children how to question and filter information, how to talk honestly, how to make assertive, conscious, independent decisions and, most importantly, how to construct a question so as to get the most effective answer from Google.

I'd love for my daughter to be able to read a magazine whilst also understanding that ninety per cent of the images are manipulated, that the models she's looking at might have sacrificed health and happiness to achieve that thigh gap, that joy isn't found in being the snazziest dresser in the room, and that great love doesn't come forth depending on how volumized your hair is (no matter how much the adverts try to pummel that message into us). At the same time, I'd love her to embrace the fun of being a woman, the joy of a buxom beehive, the buzz from a trendy neon nail, the shitty-day-quick-fix-impulse-boots purchase.

I want her to have friends that she adores and that adore her. I want her to know that her friends love her because she cares for them, and because she isn't afraid to give them kind but tough love. I want her to walk into a party and know that people are happy she is there. I want her to have that feeling about her friends. I want her to forget to shave her legs or shave them because she has chosen to or not shave her legs at all and not care for even a second – and certainly never avoid swimming or skinny-dipping (one of life's great joys) because her legs don't look like a doll's. I want her to have a body that is healthy and can facilitate everything she wants to do and everything she can't even imagine doing. I want her to dance and climb and explore and adventure and laugh and cry and not worry about whether she looks mysterious and ethereal, because not all of us can be mysterious and ethereal – some of us have to be silly and fun and sexy in our own unique way.

I want so much for her. I want the moon on a stick and the stars on a necklace but before that happens I'd like her to brush her hair and put away the paintbox like I've asked her to do three times.

The strange thing about being a parent is that your job is to teach your children how to be without you. It's my role, my responsibility, to teach them, empower them, free them and fortify them not to need me. I stop them crossing the road without looking both ways, I fold their socks, stroke their hair when they're ill, buy their favourite biscuits for their lunch boxes, take them to school, to play dates, to ballet, to kung fu, to yoghurt knitting, to the dentist – and love them so much I want to take gigantic bites out of their little bottoms – all so that I can let them go.

All I can hope for is that she wants to meet me for a bowl of pasta every so often and will feel she can cry on my shoulder whenever she needs it. I can't wait for her to grow up and at the same time I'm already sad that my little ratbag will be gone. I remember my mum once telling me that she missed her babies. I didn't really understand at the time. But now I do. Being a parent is such a surreal experience from beginning to end. Suddenly you have this tiny person who is entirely dependent on you, and then in the flicker of an eye they're independent and have transformed. Which is exactly what a parent truly wants – but it's sometimes incredibly hard.

Life is weird. People are weird. And that is great. One of my favourite Twitter pictures (so cultured, I know) is of a sign saying 'Normal people scare me'. Because we're all weird, really; the only difference between us is how good we are at concealing it. Sometimes we learn how to hide it through our upbringing or rules or religion or fear of becoming a social pariah – it's much safer to blend in than to question and expose yourself, and I have done this many, many times – but wowzers it feels good when you sense that you are around people that allow all those oddities and idiosyncrasies to come forth without the fear of being pushed away.

That is a rare and wonderful thing and if you're one of those people who embrace others regardless of their 'weirdness' then I kiss your face. Because how can people really grow without facing their true selves? And how can people acknowledge their true self if they're terrified of being bonked on the head with a ruler for being honest about it? I hope that my kids aren't cynical but instead are open and full of grace and humbleness. I hope that they know we're all, every one of us, billionaires included, one bad decision away from bankruptcy – and I hope they watch out for that sneaking sense of superiority.

Isn't it wonderful when people open themselves up and tell you something that so distinctly adds to your understanding of who they are? Don't we all, when it really comes down to it, want to understand and be understood? Isn't it amazing when you tell a close friend something you thought would freak them out and instead they respond with 'Me too!'? But I've learned that unless you are willing to lay yourself bare, people will not lay themselves bare to you. And when that happens, no one wins except the people who love rules and love everything to be neat and controlled.

But surely life is too short to pretend?

So embrace your real unfiltered self, metaphorically and physically, and embrace the people around you. Unless they've forgotten to shave their legs, obvs.

# Acknowledgements

I want to thank everyone who has helped me write this book – everyone who has kindly given their input, brought me tea and told me to stop procrastinating.

A huge thank you to Hannah for taking the time to do cringe checks and for sharing your amazing, insightful observations (such as how we often greet girls with a compliment about how they look yet with boys we simply tell them we're happy to see them, setting the message from a young age that the most important thing about a girl is her appearance. Making minor adjustments like this is how change really happens).

A huge thank you to my parents for always being so supportive, even if I'm talking about something embarrassing or taboo. Your love and open mindedness give me the freedom to be honest.

Thank you to Jenny Scott for the wonder that is Mothers Meetings. The daily connection with other women, who happen to be mothers, over Instagram, as well as actual three dimensional meetings, are such an incredible source of love, learning, energy and laughing. The inspiring entrepreneurship and camaraderie have become a fourth emergency service for me.

Thank you to my incredible agent Mary at James Grant for being the person who started this ball rolling and kept it rolling with such positivity and belief. This all started six years ago when I wrote a pitch for a book about pregnancy and, long story short, with much encouragement and after many filming-schedule battles, thanks to her it's now a real, live book. Thank you for generally being one of the most energy-giving humans I have ever met.

And thank you to wonderful Fenella at Penguin and Rowan at Furniss Lawton. Even with missed deadlines, anxious content chopping and waffling in meetings, your support and constant enthusiasm has been incredibly reassuring. From the first moment to the last you have both been unwavering in your support, so thank you. And thank you for giving your ears and (so much) time and care during very long meetings, during a very strange time in my life, when we put the world to rights and then undid it and put it back again. I hugely appreciate it.